PREFACE

There is an increased demand by the intelligent person to know more about the function of the human body. The eye is a composite structure. It is designed to point at objects and make a clear picture for the brain to analyse. The basic sciences taught at school provide sufficient knowledge to enable the average person to understand this text. The purpose of this book is to explain the overall story of the contact lens and allied devices that correct vision. There is also a short description of the use of such devices in the treatment of eye disease. This book is not intended as a textbook for those professionally engaged in contact lens practice. It may initiate the many para-medical and para-optical persons who deal with the subject and require an introduction without scientific language.

I have purposely dealt with the more mundane aspects, such as costing. The numerical examples given at these times of rapid inflation must not be quoted out of context.

I have acknowledged the several manufacturers for the use of photographs in the text. I would like to thank my secretary, Miss J. Coomber, for typing the text and my wife for acting as a lay censor.

May 1975

M.R.

CONTENTS

	Preface	iii
I	When Were Contact Lenses Invented	1
II	How the Eye Functions	6
III	How the Contact Lens Corrects Sight	21
IV	The Role of the Practitioner	27
V	Contact Lenses in Current Use	35
VI	The Fitting of the Contact Lens	41
VII	Complications	56
VIII	Use of Contact Lenses for Treatment of Eye Disease (experimental, therapeutic, diagnostic and prosthetic)	66
IX	Manufacture of Contact Lenses	72
X	Questions and Answers	80
XI	Correction of Sight by Other Methods	88
	Index	94

Chapter I

WHEN WERE CONTACT LENSES INVENTED?

From early literature and drawings we know that man has had ideas for invention far in advance of the technology available at his time. For example, Roger Bacon of the 12th century knew enough about light and images to be able to project an image on some low-lying clouds. Such ideas were the forerunners of the magic lantern of the 17th and 18th century and the modern 35-mm. automatic slide projector. The basic idea of image projection by optical image methods was essential before cinema could be developed. Certainly Leonardo da Vinci drew his notions of carriages able to travel in air, but without the knowledge of future internal combustion and electric engines and aerodynamics he was not able to consider any practical methods of lifting his air carriage. He could only use the technology of his time and designed a carriage that lifted by wings similar to those of birds. Likewise the contact lens or glass was considered by Leonardo as a feasibility but was a few centuries from the technology able to make such an invention a practicality. The observations of Descartes show that he clearly understood what happened to normal sight when a transparent fluid, such as water, came into contact with the eye. One has only to open one's eyes under water in a swimming pool to know that the ability to focus clearly has become impaired. Descartes knew this and realised that water had almost the same power to change the direction of light rays as the front of the eye. Thus the water negatived the power of the front lens of the eye. This part of the eye power is stronger than a conventional magnifying glass that can magnify by four times. He could not foresee any practical use of such phenomena. He lived at a time when many intelligent people wrote down their observations. Such collected items in the 15th and 16th century became texts of Natural Philosophy or History.

It was much later that contact glasses became of interest. About the turn of the 18th century more than one scientist became interested in the causes of eye disease. This may have coincided with the Industrial Revolution and the movement of people and large armies. At this time the ravages upon the front of the eye from malnutrition, infections, such as V.D. and trachoma, were very real. They were obvious in the large over-crowded cities and sea-ports. Thomas Young about 1812 and Herschel at about that time described small glass cups filled with fluids and jellies that could be placed on such eyes to obtain better vision. They had recognised the optical function of the front part of the eye and considered a glass cup with a spherically curved front surface as a substitute for a diseased cornea. The first half of the 19th century has many reports of similar ideas. For one particular eye disease the patient wore special spectacles which could be pushed backwards until the lens contacted the front of the eye. When this occurred good vision was obtained. But no real progress was made until man attempted to imitate the exact shape of the front of the eye.

In Germany glass blowing was highly developed and one doctor made plaster casts of the eyes and asked a glass manufacturer to make thin shells of the same shape as the eye. By trial and error very accurate copies were made. The doctor then attempted to place these glass shells on the eye. He found that the shell, if too small and thick, would not stay on the eye, so he made contact shells larger and larger until the optimum size for staying on the eye was found. Using a thickness of at least 1–2 mm. and good quality glass we know that the lenses were almost as big as the whole front of the eye, not only the part we can see between the lids but also that part under the lids.

Such lenses were approximately half a sphere in surface shape. They had no power to change the direction of light and so correct defects of sight, but eye physicians and surgeons of the later 19th century immediately understood that they could protect the eye in certain diseased states and in rare conditions even give better vision. The great firm of Zeiss and physicists, such as Abbé, took an interest in these devices. They realised that perhaps such shells could be ground into good lenses like spectacle lenses. They proved correct, and hence began an intense period of trial and error to discover how such lenses could be made. Very soon sets of lenses were manufactured by grinding methods to produce a two-curved shell: the outer curve to fit the white of the eye, and the central part to fit the cornea or glass transparent front of the eye. This was necessary because the size of the eye is very different in shape, curves and size for everyone. For example, a small-boned man from Asia has different dimensions as compared with a

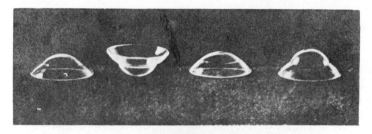

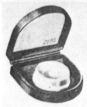

Fig. 1 A set of glass scleral contact lenses of various sizes and curves for trial fitting (circa 1920's)

large-boned Celtic Caucasian. Whilst exact fits were not possible, average shapes could be made, and the manufacturers were prepared to make in-between sizes. It was possible to fit the front of the eye by trial and error methods, combined with crude measurements by a ruler. It was furthermore understood that water must be present between the back of the lens and the eye otherwise the back of the lens steamed up and no vision was possible. The correct power could be worked out by a trial and error method, and by this tiresome and time-consuming method contact lenses to correct sight were available at the end of the last century. At that time they were considered experimental and usually not worn for more than a few hours. Patients suffered

severe blurring and redness and soreness of the eye if they
attempted more. Most patients could not wear the lenses at all.
It was discovered that many severe eye conditions gained some
vision by wearing these appliances, but they were too crude to be
applicable to all. Much thought was given to how these crude
large lenses could be improved. These advances occurred in this
century.

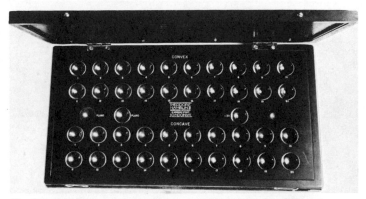

Fig. 2 Individual lenses to show shapes obtained by using different combinations of two curves and diameters.

The first advance was to apply the knowledge scientists had
obtained regarding how the front of the eye breathed, because,
to a certain extent, it does breathe, like our lungs. Putting something over the breathing surface has the same effect as occlusive
sticky plaster over the skin. The tissue underneath becomes
soggy with water and abnormal. The way contact lens advances
have, to a large extent, overcome these problems is a saga of
trial and error, science and luck. Each advance will be described
in the pages that follow in relation to the different types of lenses
and the conditions they treat.

From 1935 onwards plastics became available to the optical
industry. The public knows the name 'Perspex'. It was used in
place of windows for the domes of Spitfires and for many other
uses. Whilst the transparency is good, its softness can be a
disadvantage. The surface can become easily scratched and lose

any optical advantage is may have had. But this material can be worked by many tools, including the lathe. One cannot easily work glass, except with grinding techniques requiring long apprenticeship and experience. Furthermore, Perspex is very light in weight, but, best of all its properties, is the fact that, when heated, it becomes soft and can be moulded to other shapes. The material keeps its new shape fairly well and, since the temperature to produce such a change is only 200°C, it again wins as a material for making contact lenses. The impact of this material on contact lens practice was immediate, and great progress would have resulted had not the war intervened. After the war, large contact lenses of very thin design, copying exactly the white of the eye in shape and with perfect optical surfaces in front of the cornea, became available. A better technique of taking impressions of the eye also developed and in the 1950's we had very good methods of reproducing this shape in plastic. Such procedures would have improved had not the whole fitting of contact lenses become revolutionised by Tuohy. This optician in the States of America copied the technique of making small contact lenses that was used by 19th century workers. You will remember they failed because heavy glass would not stay on the eye if made in small sizes, but Perspex, being so light, did. Tuohy commenced with lenses 11-mm. in diameter. In the space of 20 years the optimum size for maximum tolerance was discovered. Modern small lenses in ideal circumstances can be even less than 7-mm. in diameter and 0.10-mm. thick. This is the thickness of some writing paper. Yet such a small lens can correct most people's sight!

In the middle sixties (1966) Wichterle and Lim of Czechoslovakia introduced the second innovation in this century. They found a soft wettable material which made good contact lenses. Once again, scientists and clinicians commenced to work in order to discover the best soft material and also the best size to produce lenses which, in some circumstances, can be worn constantly. This is the aim of the practitioner, to supply a lens that can, without harming the eye, be worn several weeks or months and then be changed for a new lens as easily as an item of clothing. Whilst this is the ultimate aim there is still some way to go.

Chapter II

HOW THE EYE FUNCTIONS

The eye is a ball basically about $1''$ in diameter (2.5 cm.). It is almost round except for the anterior part that has a steeper curvature. This part is no larger than a 1 penny piece (nickel): it is the front lens of the eye or the cornea. When seen from the front the eye has a white portion and a central coloured part called the iris. The iris has a round opening at its centre called the pupil. Behind the pupil is a small lens, which is almost round in shape and half the size of the eye, with water in front of the lens and jelly behind. The back of the eye has a pigmented blood vessel layer and in front of this a thin transparent nerve layer, which is called the retina. The whole eye can be likened to a camera. Imagine a ball-shaped camera with its lenses in front and the curved film or retina at the back. The iris in the camera is the aperture, which can be altered to give different size pupils. The pupil of the eye works automatically. If the light increases, the pupil becomes smaller. A camera works in exactly the same way. Those cameras fitted with electronic devices do this automatically, otherwise one would have to look up tables and calculate distances, lighting and aperture size according to the sensitivity of the film. The human eye takes into account all such calculations, either chemically in the tissues or by nerves and cell reflexes in the brain. It is a complicated and well-balanced system. If any part goes wrong, the individual becomes visually inconvenienced.

Light from the sun illuminates objects several thousand times more brightly than electric light, yet we unconsciously can change our retina sensitivity in a matter of minutes. It is as though one could change the sensitivity of a photo film from 10 ASA to 100 ASA almost instantly, but one must remember that it can sometimes take $\frac{1}{2}$-hour to get used to very dark surroundings. This is due to the chemicals responsible for the function of

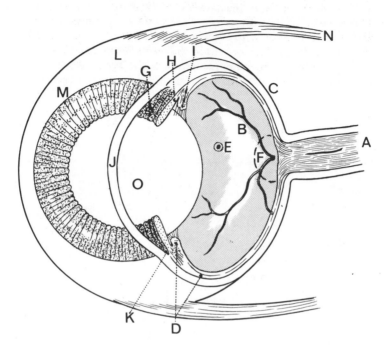

Fig. 3 Three dimensional drawing

  A Optic nerve
  B Retinal Artery
  C Outer Tissue of Eye (Sclera)
  D Ciliary body and Choroid
  E Centre of Sight – Fovea
  F Optic Nerve Exit from eye
  G Iris
  H Ciliary Muscle
  I Part of Muscle used to accommodate lens of eye
  J Cornea
  K Drainage Angle of Eye
  L Sclera or White Coat
  M Rim of Cornea
  N Outside Muscle of Eye
  O Lens of Eye

the low-illumination retina having to undergo several processes before being sufficiently active to work. We are essentially a day animal and we work with the whole of the retina. Under daylight conditions the millions of cells in the retina respond with different intensities, depending upon the nature of the light. Thus most of the cells are concerned just with responding to light, irrespective

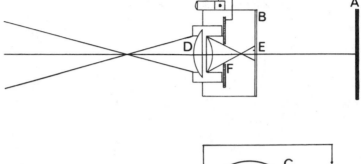

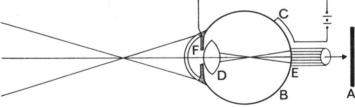

Fig. 4 The eye is like a camera
- A. The printed and developed picture at the brain
- B. The film or retina
- C. The photo electric cell that controls the aperture of the camera or the nerve reflex that controls the pupil of the eye.
- D. The lens.
- E. The image
- F. The aperture or pupil.

of its colour, and for this crude sensitivity groups of cells work together. Others work singly and are mostly found at the centre of sight. This area resembles the small round hole at the centre of a radar bowl. This centre is concerned with receiving focussed images and colour sense.   At night when the light is very poor, the cells outside this centre, which are concerned mostly with light and not colour, become more highly activated or adapted. Thus man can get round at night with very poor lighting and also using the same basic equipment adapt and accommodate to bright daylight.

For contact lenses the front of the eye is our main concern. The lens will be touching many areas of the front of the eye. It is important to know how the contact lens can be made to fit and what changes may arise from wearing the lens. In order to

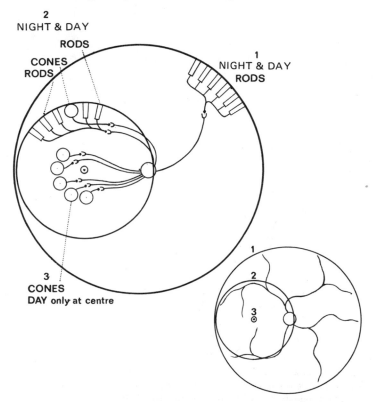

Fig. 5 The three areas of distribution for the cells that receive light
1. Periphery – Rods can adapt for night vision.
2. Equator and around Fovea – For day and night adaptation
3. Fovea at centre for adaptation to bright light, such as day-time.

understand these problems, we must describe how the cornea functions.

The Cornea

This is the window of the eye. It is about 1-mm. thick at the edge where it joins the white of the eye and half that thickness at the centre. Providing the surface is wet and kept so by blinking, the cornea remains transparent. It has a curvature which is almost

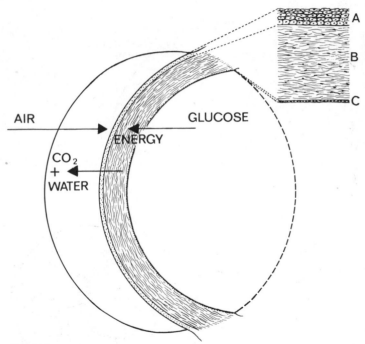

Fig. 6 The Cornea
The surface cells require oxygen and glucose and water to function.
The end-products are carbon dioxide, gas and water.
The cornea consists of
    A = Surface Cells (epithelium)
    B = Tough Interlacing Fibres (Stroma)
    C = Inside cells which keep the cornea transparent.

spherical at the centre. Throughout our lives the front surface
layer of cells of the cornea are being replaced, and they grow and
die at a high rate. Some cells that die just dissolve away and form
chemicals which can be removed by tear fluids or via inside and
outside tissues of the eye. Some cells die with a debris that is
collected by the lids' blinking action into a deposit that is often

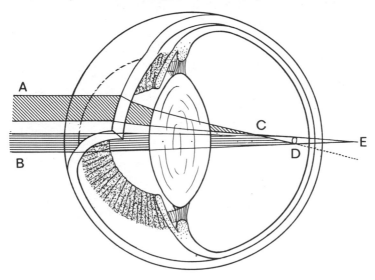

Fig. 7 Optical Pathway
The light has been divided into two pathways
    A = Beam in the vertical, and
    B = Beam in the horizontal
The astigmatism of the eye produces two images at C and E (line images).
The area of image at D is for the normal eye at the fovea.

wiped from the eye. To regenerate the cells oxygen is required
and also various foods, such as glucose and proteins. Such foods
are brought to the eye from the blood stream, but because the
cornea is transparent and has no blood vessels the final part of
the journey has to be made either through the eye or over its
surface. Without oxygen the process is slowed down or stopped.
Without oxygen, even if the regeneration of cells continues, the
side products can prove harmful to the cornea. Fortunately the eye

can do without oxygen for short periods and certainly perform most of its functions when the oxygen is very low. Furthermore, when the lids are closed, the oxygen is low anyway, so the eye is well used to maintaining normality with low oxygen levels.

The curvature of the cornea determines two-thirds of the total optical power of the eye. The power to which I refer is that able to bend the rays of light from any object in front of the eye. The

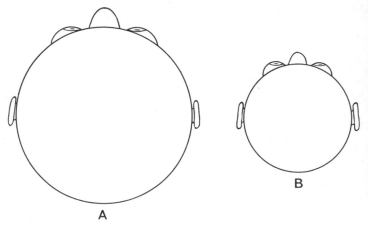

Fig. 8 Eye Size
The larger the head the larger the eye and the flatter the curvatures of the surface.

bending of the rays of light ultimately forms a focus or image at the retina. Therefore the power, quality of surface and the transparency of the cornea are important. The normal eye is not the same size for everyone. Depending upon the size of the head, so will the corneal size and curves vary. A small head has steeper curved cornea and usually a smaller eye. Conversely a man with a large head has a larger eye and also a flatter curve of the cornea. Some races who are small-boned will have steeper corneal curves. Women will have steeper curved and smaller eyes than men of the same ethnic group. One would expect babies and children to have smaller eyes and steeper corneas. In fact, they do, but since the head of a baby is large when compared with its body the cornea is only very little different from the adult.

Types of Variation in Eye Power

As the child grows the eye power changes to keep pace with the changing length of the eye. To return to the analogy of the camera, if the lens power in the camera is too weak, then the image will be formed behind the film. If the body of the camera can be lengthened, then the image can be made to form a clear picture on the film. Alternatively, one could change the lens for a stronger one and achieve the same effect. The human eye can naturally make some changes to correct the vision. The changes are mainly concerned with adding power. Thus in young people the lens in the eye can add power almost up to a third of its total. This means that if the eye is shorter or if the power of the eye is less than it should be, the extra can be made up by changing the power of the lens in the eye. Unfortunately the ability to change power gradually decreases and almost disappears by the age of 60. The type of vision error where the focus or image forms behind the eye is known as long-sighted. Theoretically such patients can only see well in the distance and not for near. The opposite is know as short-sight. This means that the image is formed in front of the back of the eye. Either because the power of the eye is too strong or the eye too big and long, short-sighted eyes can see well at near but poorly at long distances. Unfortunately there is no known mechanism for nature to correct this type of sight. The lens in the eye cannot become weaker by even 1/60th of the total power. Therefore all short-sight has to be corrected by artificial methods, such as spectacles or contact lenses.

The personality and function of individuals is often related to their ability to see well. For example, in infancy good vision is not necessary since survival is in the hands of the parent. The infant can find out most details of their immediate environment by touch and smell. Vision provides just the outline of objects at that age. By the age of 2 the vision is much improved and almost good enough to pass the driving test, i.e. see a registration number plate in daylight at 25 yards. Furthermore, the infant can now change his focus from distance to near. This automatic device has enabled man to develop both as a hunter and a craftsman. In many animals there is a natural pre-emption for either good near or far, but rarely both. The eye that cannot do these things we classify as abnormal. From the contact lens point of view, it is mostly the errors of optical power that can be corrected. These are an interesting group of conditions that account for the majority of power errors in the human eye.

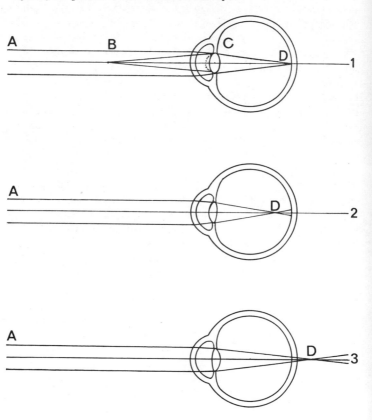

Fig. 9 The focus and the retina
  1. Distance Light + Normal eye = Clear image (D)
      (A)
      For near object B the eye changes its power at C (Lens accommodation)
  2. Distance Light + Short-sighted eye (Myopia) = Blurred Image
  3. Distance Light + Long-sighted eye = Blurred Image

If the window to the eye (cornea) becomes scarred from disease or development, then good sight may not be possible. Spectacles will not help. If the scarring affects the centre few millimetres of the window, then very poor vision can result. We will describe later how the contact lens can help even this type of eye problem.

The vast majority of eye disorders are in reality variations about the normal. One must expect at least 85% of eyes to develop normally, but in the remainder the exact power and positions of the various parts of the eye are not quite right. This does not mean that the eye is diseased, any more than your foot is diseased if you require size $6\frac{1}{2}$ or 10 in shoes when the average size is 8 (men). The diagram (Fig. 9) shows each part of the eye and how even a tenth part of a millimetre change in position or radius of curvature will alter the position of the image. Thus if the image falls in front of the back of the eye it is known as myopia and hypermetropia when behind. This is supposing this error to be the same in each meridian of the eye. It is common for the eye to show a variation in powers; there may be normal vision in the horizontal axis but slight short-sight in the vertical. This type of error is known as astigmatism (Fig. 7). We all posess a little astigmatism and it does not affect our sight, but if the difference in power is great then we are advised to correct our sight. Some people discover that by screwing the lids together and seeing through a narrow chink between the lids the sight does improve. To do this occasionally is not harmful, but to attempt this all the time can be harmful, tiring and lead to headaches. If this type of defect belongs to the front surface of the eye, then a contact lens will correct the sight almost every time, sometimes better than spectacles. We will also see that when astigmatic error comes from within the eye special contact lenses are necessary. Ordinary contact lenses will then not fully correct the sight. It must be realised that for most low forms of astigmatism spectacles can often fully correct the sight.

The Lens of the Eye

Whilst it is true that the front window of the eye is the most powerful part of the eye but from a focusing point of view, it is fixed and unchangeable. The human eye, when young, must be able to change its focus. This ability to change the focus belongs to a small lens which is situated just behind the iris and in front of the very centre point of the eye. It is shaped like a lentil and

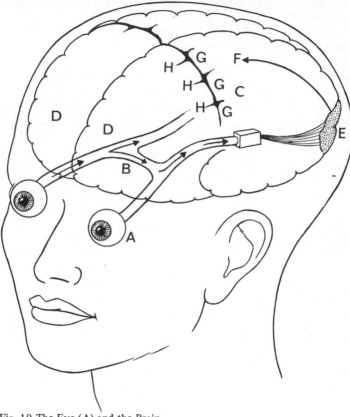

Fig. 10 The Eye (A) and the Brain
The optic nerves partly cross (B) over, so that both sides of the brain are used.

D = Front of Brain (?memory)
C = Middle Brain (judgment, etc.)
E = Back Brain (for sight)
H = Centres initiating movement in body
G = Centres receiving sensation

about half the size of your little finger-nail in diameter. Such a lens can change its curvatures. Thus, when looking in the distance, the front surface is relatively flat, but when looking near to, the front surface becomes steeper. This changing of power occurs unconsciously in the normal eye. Gradually as the tissue within the lens becomes harder this power of accommodating to different distances is lost, so that most people of 40 and over need some optical help for near work.

The long-sighted individual has to use some of the focusing power to correct his sight for distance. So he is at a further disadvantage when it comes to near work, since he may not have enough focusing power left. Thus some people require help for reading, even when young, when they have a high degree of longsight. Short-sighted people have good near sight without help from spectacles or contact lenses. They do not use the focusing lens inside the eye as much as the normal. We will see later that for contact lens wearers this can be a disadvantage.

When the lens inside the eye becomes diseased and opaque, it is seen in the pupil of the eye as white or grey. Normally we cannot see a person's internal lens of the eye.

The eye, therefore, has an optical system made of soft transparent tissues. In life the pressure of fluids within the eye keeps the outside tissues of the eye and, of course, the cornea quite rigid. This permits good optical surfaces to be maintained. One must ask how good is the best eye's performance when compared with man-made optical instruments.

The eye is not designed as an optical instrument in isolation. It has developed its peculiar optical system with all its faults in conjunction with the retina and the brain. It would be wasteful for nature to develop a more elaborate optical system for the eye capable of reducing colour aberrations and optical distortions when the retina and brain are unable to appreciate these sophistications. Therefore one finds that the human animal is designed to discriminate for the distance two stars in the sky if they are at an angle of 40' to the eye. When this is applied to near objects one can read print when the height of a letter is 1 mm.

These statements are only true if the illumination is sufficient to stimulate the most critical and sensitive part of our central vision of the retinae.

Irrespective of how good the eye is, the sensation of sight ultimately depends upon the brain. The messages from the eye are interpreted by the brain and eventually reach a level of perception. This may work by a subconscious system of comparison between the immediate received image picture and the millions of other pictures that have been stored or memorised in complicated patterns of recognition. It is indeed very complex, and by comparison a modern computer is simple. Even the personality and environment of the individual can affect visual perception.

One must conclude that for the normal eye, whilst the optical system may only be half as good as a modern instrument, it is for its size and function a very adequate instrument.

Fortunately we have two eyes. Apart from having one in reserve, the use of two eyes is to form two pictures and cover a larger area or field of view. Because the eyes are some 6 to 7 cms. apart, the two pictures formed of one object are very slightly different. The two pictures received by the brain can only be easily fused into one by subconsciously inhibiting and highlighting parts of the picture. The total result is a projected tilting of the picture in space. What the individual sees in his imagination is not a flat picture but a picture in depth. We call this stereoscopic vision. Some individuals have a 'stereoscopic' depth of vision using one eye only. They are people who for some reason have been unable to develop the use of two eyes together from an early age.

Contact lenses have several functions to play, apart from correcting vision. This is but the beginning. They have to determine field of vision and also maintain stereoscopic vision, otherwise they fail. The sense of vision does not work in isolation, it works with all our other senses. Thus hearing, balance, smell, even taste and touch, play a part with sight in making the human animal alert and in positive health. By giving an individual normal sight, the other senses can work to a different level. The personality of an individual is greatly affected by the stimuli that come to the brain from all his senses. If they are correctly balanced, the result is more likely to be a normal mentally and physically balanced human-being. We know that if the young child who has had sight is suddenly deprived of this faculty he becomes silent and withdrawn. For some days they may curl up and wish to go

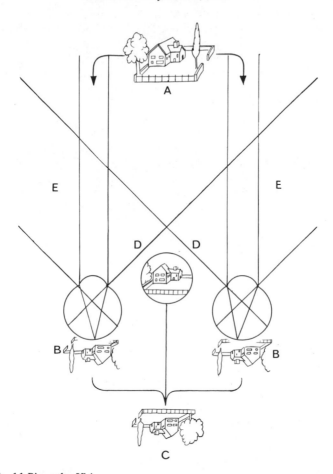

Fig. 11 Binocular Vision
Two separate images fuse in the brain to form one upside down picture
simulating depth (stereoscopic vision)

    A = The object
    ED= Limits of Fields of Vision
    B = Image formed at the Retina
    C = Inverted Fused Image

to sleep until they mentally can compensate with the world through their other normal senses. The young adult who is gradually losing sight undergoes periods of increasing frustration, wishing to do so many things requiring vision but continually failing. Repetitive failure can be very depressing and leads some humans to over-compensate. They do develop activities commensurate with their other senses. This can have good results. For example, the short-sighted individual becomes a bookworm and not a sportsman. The sense of hearing may be developed to include music and even the playing of an instrument. On the other hand, some may opt out of society or education and take up less desirable roles.

The giving of normal vision is important. One must remember that so far man has attempted to solve the problem by peripheral appliances but the future may determine other techniques of ensuring that normal vision is for everyone.

Chapter III

HOW THE CONTACT LENS CORRECTS SIGHT

It is not my intention to use the physics of light in order to explain how a contact lens works, but if one can imagine that with a contact lens the eye has two front layers: that is a double cornea. Providing the double cornea was made of the same material, then the front surface of the first cornea (contact lens) would be chiefly responsible for bending the rays of light. Providing the front surface of the contact lens was of the correct curvature for the sight of the eye, then a clear picture would be focused on the back of the eye. A contact lens made of human cornea is the ideal contact lens. Unfortunately there is not an unlimited amount of cornea going abegging from which one can make such contact lenses. Technically we can cut cornea to different curvatures, but such a cornea-contact lens would degenerate and die after about one month. Therefore we have developed other materials which can take the place of this ideal. The materials chiefly used are polymethyl methacrylate or Medical Perspex, water absorbing acrylates and silicone rubber. These materials have different physical, chemical and optical properties. We must describe these first since they will help us to understand how they function.

Polymethyl methacrylate — Medical Perspex

This is a very light material in weight. A small contact lens need weigh only 14 mg. (milligrammes). The effect of gravity on such a lens is minimal and if the fluid film behind the lens is sufficiently sticky and the fitting correct, it will stay on the eye in a central position. The lids will disturb the fit and so will eye movement. Likewise ventilation, temperature and sudden watering of the eye will disturb the centring of a lens. These remarks apply to a different degree to all contact lenses. Medical Perspex transmits almost all natural light, even ultraviolet. This may be considered as a disadvantage. Too bright an image can disturb some patients. Therefore many lenses are tinted. This material can be tinted by several dyes, or by suspensions of inert material in the substance. The front surface of the lens can furthermore be coloured by spraying on a tinted material. Powdered charcoal is one method of tinting the material, but too much makes the material porous and difficult to use for thin lenses.

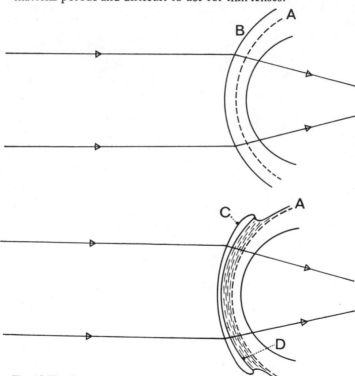

Fig. 12 The Contact Lens on the Eye
1. If the contact were made of the same material as the cornea
2. The contact lens system
    C. Contact Lens
    D. Tear Fluid
  A. – – – In both cases the front of the eye loses its power
at the corneal surface.

Perspex will melt at 200°C and can be used either in powder or sheet form to mould to different shapes. After manufacture the lens is used at normal body temperature but, even boiling will not change its shape. Imperfections result from heating and rapidly cooling impure materials and pressure on plastic will also affect its transparency. For example, the cooling of the material after it has flowed or been pressed onto a mould, in some people's opinion, should be slow. This problem, called annealing, goes on for a long time. In other manufacturers' opinions, it should be rapidly cooled so as to set the molecules and produce a stabile shape. The latter technique can produce stress in the material. This means that zones of weakness are present and can result in areas of optical imperfection or even breakage.

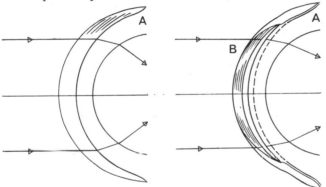

Fig. 13 The bending of light by the cornea (left) and the new system when a contact lens is worn.

This material can absorb small amounts of water and it takes several weeks for the material to reach a state of equilibrium with water when totally immersed. Therefore a thin contact lens is likely to absorb its total water quicker than a block of material. In practice, the polished surface of the material appears difficult to wet. It is only when one adds substances that make water stickier that a film can be formed over the material. We will later realise how important the property of wetting surfaces is for the contact lens and the eye. At this time polymethyl methacrylate is without doubt the cheapest and easiest material from which contact lenses can be made.

Water-absorbing Plastics (Hydrophilic Gels)

The chemistry of plastics is quite involved. Whilst many materials depend upon a regular pattern for their molecules, others form quite the contrary — an irregular pattern. Crystals are an example of molecular forces with strong linkages, so that molecules join together in a definite pattern always the same in a particular environment and built up in three dimensional forms. When the molecules are long and thin, they often become interwoven and when the environment is right they gel into a position. Sometimes the sides of the molecules become attached to each other, so forming stronger links. The molecular bricks do not always build up into a geometrical form but sometimes an amorphous and loose form. The gel state is consistent with the sudden resolving of the molecular pattern from loose chains to relatively fixed chains. Often great heat is expended whilst the process is going on. One speaks of the end result as a polymer. The polymer can consist of molecules of the same type or of different types (copolymers). Polymers in nature are extremely common and most of our body tissue consists of this form of chemistry. Many polymers are in a state which can change. Thus light and sound radiations can reverse the polymer to single loose molecular state (monomers). Some of these monomers are vapours and when they have left the material leave zones of weakness. The materials from which contact lenses are made are therefore not stabile in the same sense as metals. Polymers made from copolymers tend to be less stabile than those from single monomers.

One knows that gelatin, when dry, can exist in dry brittle sheets or powder. Likewise many of these high water-absorbing polymers appear very hard when dry but, on taking up water, become much larger and, in some instances, very soft. There is now available a series of materials which are hydrophilic acrylates. They can be manufactured by cutting the material with lathes or by moulding, and can produce lenses so soft that they are unable to keep their shape in air.

The other material worth mentioning is silicon rubber. At this time there is no successful lens but with research proceeding at such a fast rate there could well be good lenses in a few years. This material is very much like rubber but transparent. It has one very attractive property in which it excels. This is the ability to allow almost free passage of gases. Oxygen can get through such a lens to the eye. At this time the manufacturing process is not perfected and the public have only tried experimental lenses.

We shall see that all materials have specialised uses in the treatment of eye disorders. The opening paragraph stated the ideal. This was a material of the same light-bending power as the human eye. When such a lens was placed on the eye, the back surface assumed a perfect fit and there was optical continuity between the lens and eye. The front surface of the lens became the new front of the eye and to this man could give any curvature he wished so as to produce normal sight.

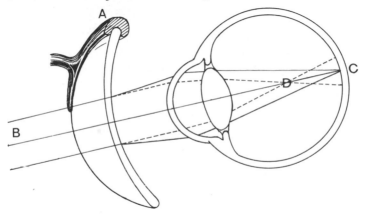

Fig. 14 The spectacle lens correcting the sight of short-sight (myopia).

Unfortunately all the materials used at this time have a bending light power (B.L.P.) higher than the eye. If the material is soft or if the back surface is exactly the same as the eye, then the problem is simplified. The surface separating the eye from the lens has a power approximately one-third of the normal cornea. The front surface, therefore, has to provide the remaining two-thirds plus or minus, whatever is required to correct the sight. The problem is slightly more complex for a lens that does not follow the curvature of the front surface of the eye. Thus when the front surface of the lens is flatter than the eye, a minus power effect is produced and vice versa when the back surface of the lens is steeper. There is a limit to what advantage such effects can produce since the back surface must, whenever possible, be a good fit. These limitations will be discussed in the next chapter.

The patient often asks the practitioner how the spectacle lens power is related to the contact lens. If the spectacle lens could be pushed back until it touched the cornea and, at the same time, the size shrink until it fitted the eye, then the spectacle lens has become a contact lens. The same power is not required. Thus, as the short-sighted spectacle correction approaches the eye, less power is required and vice versa for long sight.

To sum up — the contact lens increases the length of the eye and introduces a higher B.L.P. The power required to correct the sight is determined by the shape and form of the lens. For most contact lenses the back surfaces conform to the shape of the cornea whilst the front surface determines the power.

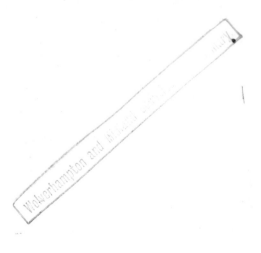

Chapter IV

THE ROLE OF THE PRACTITIONER

The contact lens is an appliance to correct sight and/or treat
eye disease. The practitioner's role must be, in the first instance,
to assess the need. If there is a case for using such an aid, then
the second stage must be to determine the feasibility. The next
step will be the fitting procedure, itself, with the measuring of
the eye and sight. Once the contact lens has been made and fitted
to the practitioner's satisfaction, the patient then begins to learn
how to use the lens. During the period of adaptation the practitioner must re-assess the appliance and measurements as need be,
so that the maximum tolerance for each individual is achieved in
optimum time. Thereafter the after-care resolves into maintenance
of the lens at its maximum performance; observation of the eye
to avoid and, when necessary, to treat complications secondary
to contact lens wear as they arise.

This chapter will deal with the several practitioners involved
in contact lens practice. It will describe their background, mode
of practice and ethics. This will permit the patient to orientate
himself as to his best procedure for seeking advice in this subject.

If a contact lens wearer is asked some years later where they
obtained their contact lenses the answers can be very varied. One
may say 'I was in Hong Kong for 48 hours and I know they are
cheap there, so I went to the first shop advertising lenses and
obtained them the same day.' The same remarks may be made
regarding some German lenses. One patient stated that a certain
well-known optician in Germany sold and supplied lenses the
same day and with a cheap return flight from London the total
cost was less than lenses obtained in London. If price is to be the
only criterion and contact lenses are to be considered as a commodity and not a service, then by all means shop around until you
find the cheapest deal. This attitude has been voiced by responsible
journalists and T.V. interviewers who should know better. The

simple truth is that contact lenses are not a commodity but more a service; that whilst several forms and materials are available the service required of the practitioner is more important than the commodity. If, at any time in the future, the lens becomes uniform in fitting and material, then the service component will decrease. Since the cost of the lens is fairly uniform, the extra cost of professional services makes up the variable fees quoted for fitting and supplying contact lenses. The purpose of this chapter will be to explain why practitioners set different scales of payment on their services and also explain how the National Health Service is involved.

The basic material is manufactured by plastics chemists. The biggest chemical plants may be involved in the production of such materials, but since the amount required is small, it is not impossible for an individual technician or plastics chemist to produce sufficient material for thousands of lenses in a room not larger than 10$'$ × 10$'$ with equipment costing £1,500 ($ 3000) Many small laboratories exist throughout the world, some in association with manufacturers of lenses, others by themselves. The advancement of the science of plastics technology will in the larger concerns be programmed and money set aside for research. The research into materials and manufacture is chiefly in the hands of industry, but occasionally the academic scientist becomes involved. Because there is a world-wide demand for better contact lenses and because they have a profit margin, there is a stimulus at the material stage. This is essential if contact lenses are to advance. One hopes that even more money will be spent in future to develop new and better materials. When we discuss the problems with present lenses and materials, it will readily be understood where future research should be directed.

The basic ingredients required to make the plastic are not expensive when purchased in bulk, but one must realise that with research and development, control of quality, and the usual overheads, even mass-production can result in an expensive piece of plastic.   The basic plastic end product may cost anything from £1 to £3 (2 to 6 dollars). The end product produced by the plastics chemist will be a circular thick button no larger than a coat button and $\frac{1}{4}''$ thick. When thousands of buttons are required each week by a small manufacturing laboratory, there is an irresistable desire to employ a technician and make one's own plastic. Whilst this is sound economy, it does not help further the research and development programmes of large plastic chemical laboratories.

The better plastic chemists take a lively interest in the clinical aspects of contact lens practice. They are often members of contact lens societies and discuss the subject at some depth with clinicians. These industrial scientists have contributed much to the development of contact lens practice, but, being a new entry to the scene, their motives are often held suspect by the more conservative practitioners.

The manufacturer is a species of practitioner who comes from all walks of life. Accountants become manufacturers. Doctors and opticians, especially in Japan, are often involved in manufacture. In some instances they become solely concerned with manufacture and do not engage in clinical practice. Certainly many engineers have become manufacturers and with their expert knowledge of lathes and tooling are ideally suited for this role. They, too, are vitally interested in the clinical progress of the contact lens wearing patient. Therefore as with any other clinical sciences team-work is essential for high standards of practice.

The ophthalmic surgeon or ophthalmologist is a medical practitioner who specialises in the diagnosis and treatment of the eye diseases. The role of this practitioner varies according to basic training, qualifications, hospital and university appointments and even interests of the particular practitioner. Several ophthalmologists are interested in the abnormalities of the eye which are considered within normal physiological limits and their correction. They are therefore particularly interested in the way contact lenses can be used for their treatment. But of especial importance is the interest ophthalmologists have in the contact lens changes to eye tissue and their use in serious eye diseases. Furthermore, their use to correct eye power problems that result from eye operations or their use in operations are of particular interest. In Chapter VIII a description of such eye problems will be given. The time given in the training of the ophthalmic surgeon to sight-testing and optometric measurement is small when compared with the whole period of specialist training. Likewise it is not uncommon for a trained ophthalmologist to know very little about the mechanics of contact lens fitting, since optical dispensing procedures are not included in the courses. This does not apply to the larger centres of training, but there are almost in every country and especially in the U.S.A. and upon the continent of Europe an increasing number of ophthalmologists who may be as well trained as optometrists in these matters and, of course, have as well a vast amount of knowledge stemming from general medicine and surgery. On top of this they have the knowledge of ophthalmic medicine and surgery. This helps balance the levels of practitioners available to the patient. It also explains the fee differential between ophthalmologist and optician. Whilst in a free society the services of a qualified ophthalmologist who specialises in contact lens practice are available to all who can afford the fee, this is not a good use of professional manpower. Society must make best use of its trained professional manpower. Thus it would seem morally wrong to encourage medical specialists to spend most of their professional lifetime doing sight-testing and contact lens fitting on normal individuals when there exists a large body of well-trained opticians able to do the same work. In some countries this is not the case. The public, if offered the choice of practitioners for contact lens fitting, must realise that the professional services of an ophthalmologist will make the purchase of contact lenses sometimes twice that of an optician. The reasons for requiring an ophthalmologist's services are always if eye abnormality exists or when eye disease secondary or with association of contact lens wear occurs. The follow-up of the eye health by an ophthalmologist will be done obviously by an individual experienced in diagnosis of eye disease whereas the optician has been taught essentially in the measurement of eye normality and the recognition but not diagnosis of eye abnormality.

The present-day optician has developed from the seller of spectacles and optical instruments. In many countries university courses exist to train optometrists. They are a profession who have developed from the optician, but are now more concerned with the examination of vision and the eye. They are trained to recognise abnormality but not to diagnose and treat eye disease. If they do so, it may be considered an offence in some countries. They have had a lengthy training in optics, testing of sight and contact lens practice. In some communities they must not practise in shop premises. This is to differentiate them from the dispensing optician who works from a shop. The latter can also fit contact lenses but in the U.K. must only do so at the discretion or under the supervision of an ophthalmologist or ophthalmic optician. The ophthalmic optician is the analogous U.K. professional man to the optometrist. But there are no laws preventing the ophthalmic optician practising from shop premises. Indeed one may also find medical specialist ophthalmic practitioners also practising from shop premises in the U.K. At some future time both types of practitioner will leave shop premises and practise solely from clinics or consulting rooms.

The patient seeking contact lenses has the dilemma of choosing a practitioner who may be one of three separate professions — the ophthalmologist, the ophthalmic optician (optometrist) and the dispensing optician. Furthermore, there is the added problem that some opticians may possess contact lens practice diplomas and others none. The ophthalmologist who ethically will only see a patient referred by a medical practitioner and may not be interested in contact lens practice, but he may employ a technician who does this work. The problem is not so real as indicated since there is a chain of reference. The few ophthalmologists who specialise in contact lens practice are known by other ophthalmologists or by dispensing opticians. The opticians, both dispensing and ophthalmic, are allowed to advertise their expertise discreetly in their shop windows or letter headings. An advertisement that is overt or over-zealous must be considered non-ethical, even though no disciplinary action is taken by the General Optical Council.

Once the patient has made a choice of practitioner, whether it be an individual choice or by referral, the procedure is usually as follows: The patient attends for a consultation with spectacle prescription if available, or certainly their spectacles or present contact lenses (if worn). The practitioner will take a full history, including some details of general illnesses that can affect the eye and vision. Such a history will often include questions regarding tablets, pills or other treatment the patient is having from a medical practitioner. This information need not be given if the practitioner is non-medical, but such information, if given, will help all contact lens practitioners in the management of problems likely to subsequently arise.

If the patient is in doubt the contact lens practitioner should be asked to communicate with the patient's medical practitioner for further details. For example, if a patient has diabetes of long standing, there are certain well-known eye complications that can occur. It is as well that the contact lens practitioner knows that there is the complication of diabetes, so that the eye tissues can be examined periodically and any contact lens complications be correctly assessed. If a female patient is on the contraceptive pill, is pregnant or suffers from anaemia it is also wise to inform the practitioner, since again certain problems may become manifest with contact lens wear.

Whilst the role of the dispenser optician may be limited to the contact lens fitting, he is usually supplied with information regarding acuity, so that the best possible correction can be given. If an eye with disease is being fitted, then it is imperative that the lens be fitted by or with the closest supervision of the ophthalmologist.

The ophthalmic optician or optometrist will be able to do vision and eye measurements necessary for contact lens fitting. Contact lens practice is often considered by many opticians as a speciality. Some, therefore, work in consulting rooms as do medical specialists. The patient must not be confused as to the role of optician practitioner. They are not ophthalmologists or medical specialists and will not attempt to diagnose or treat eye disease. If the patient has an eye disease which has had treatment or is being treated, then it is imperative they let the contact lens practitioner know, irrespective of his professional status. Failure to do so could affect the type of lens to be fitted and the after-care management.

If the patient chooses to consult an ophthalmic optician for contact lenses and, as a result of the first examination, there is some doubt concerning the health of the eye, then the ophthalmic optician will almost always refer the patient to an ophthalmologist for advice before proceeding with the contact lens fitting.

It is usual for any practitioner to discuss the question of fees regarding contact lenses at the first consultation. In some practices the fees are discussed by the receptionist or secretary. The patient must remember that the basic contact lens material is inexpensive, but the professional and technical time and know-how and the research and development costs represent the major part of the fee. The following breakdown of a contact lens charge may prove helpful.

For each patient:

(4 buttons of material @ 50p. each ($ 1)	£2.00)	$ (4)
Manufacturer's price for lenses (average)	£20.00	” 40
No. of principal consultations = 3		
If ophthalmic surgeon	(£30.00)	” (60)
If ophthalmic optician	(£15.00)	” (30)
No. of technical consultations = 4	£12.00	” 24
	£47 – £62.00	$ 94–124

This fee excludes any additional requirements, such as lens case, solutions, asepticisation equipment, or indeed the overheads of the practitioner. The latter will be high for West-end practice. For contact lens practice done in clinics with manufacturing laboratories on the premises, it will be lowest. It is not unknown for such set-ups to be able to lower the cost of the lenses, so that even fees of £35 or less have been charged. Such clinics are being subsidised by the manufacturer.

Low fees do not necessarily mean an inferior contact lens but could mean less experienced practitioners and often a change of practitioner almost at every visit.

Patients often ask why they cannot obtain contact lenses under the N.H.S. In fact, they can, but the decision to supply lenses paid by the Hospital Management Committee rests with the Consultant Ophthalmic Surgeon appointed to a hospital. The referral of a patient to such a clinic must be by arrangement with a medical practitioner. In most instances a contact lens will only be prescribed if it is a clinical necessity. This means the contact lens is required in preference to spectacle lenses for better vision or is a treatment of the eye itself when suffering from disease.

The ophthalmic services of the U.K. provide spectacles but not contact lenses. If at any time a scheme could be worked out that would permit the patient to be fitted at little extra cost to the Health Service than with spectacles then the contact lens might be offered as an alternative.

Chapter V

CONTACT LENSES IN CURRENT USE

Contact lenses can be classified as to size and shape and secondly as to material. Almost all shapes and sizes can be obtained in a variety of materials.

Scleral or Haptic

These lenses can be divided into three parts for the purpose of description: the centre for sight (optical), the outside part for fitting the globe of the eye and the part in between is a smooth slope or blend from one part of steep curvature to the other of flatter curvature.

The lens may have to be filled with physiological fluid before being inserted since if air becomes locked between the centre and the cornea good vision will not be possible.

The centre part can be coloured to reduce glare of bright light. It can be painted to give the iris a different colour or act as an artificial iris if it is absent for any reason. Likewise the haptic part can be coloured white. The inside of the lens can be painted black to stop light entering the eye either totally or in part. This can be done to stop double vision problems.

Modifications to the basic fitting are:

(1) Grooves or channels made in the inside surface of the haptic to permit greater flow of tear fluid.

(2) Holes made at the transition area to allow air to form around but not over the centre of the cornea.

The purpose of these modifications is to increase the wearing time if lack of oxygen seriously affects sight and the health of the eye.

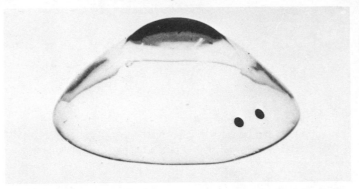

Fig. 15 Scleral hard lens — made from an impression of the eye.

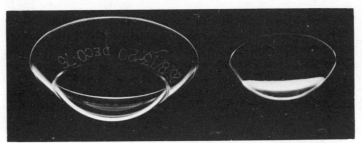

Fig. 16 Scleral hard lens made with a lathe with spherical curves.

Use of Scleral Lens

Advantages   For eyes and sight where other lenses cannot be fitted.

For shell and lens prosthetics.

For lenses required to give stable vision for short periods.

For very dry eyes.

For appliances for diagnosis of sight and electrical energy, etc.

For very active sports.

Contraindications
        Constant wear not advised.
        Distorts the eye if badly fitted.
        Fitting takes several weeks and tolerance poor for
          the average eye.

Material   Can be made in glass or hard plastic. In modified
        form in softer plastics.

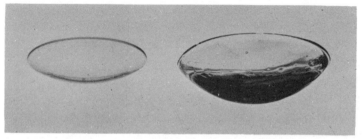

Fig. 17 Small thin hard corneal lens compared with Hydrophilic (gel) soft lens.

Intermediate or Corneo-Scleral Lenses

These lenses are between 12 and 18 mm. in size. They have either one or more back curves to permit the lens to just touch the apex of the cornea, but chiefly bear upon the white of the eye. They are useful for almost all the conditions for which scleral or haptic lenses were used. If made of hard materials several fittings are necessary, and they have to be made very thin to be worn by the normal eye. This type of lens is most commonly made in softer materials and worn very successfully by the normal and abnormal eye.

It is made, therefore, in several materials. Some are even softer than normal eye tissue. For normal degrees of softness (twice as hard as eye tissue) one or more curves are used on the back surface of the lens, but for very soft materials a conoidal or one spherical curve is all that is necessary. The very thin lenses are best for tolerance, but they break easily and do not last a long

LOW POWER SOFT LENS 13mm to 17mm

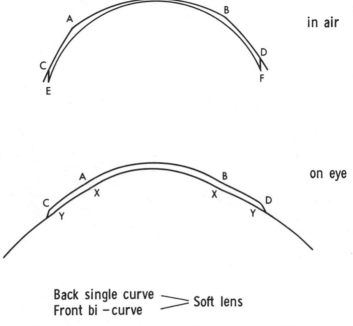

Fig. 18 To show how a soft lens takes on the curve of the eye.

time. They have the greatest use in aphakia (after cataract removal) and after graft operations when hard materials are used.
When soft materials are used, the correction of sight can be
best vision are often necessary. Astigmatic corrections can now be
added to some soft lenses.

Corneal Lenses

Sometimes called micro-corneal or by a manufacturer's trade
name.

All corneal lenses are the same size or smaller than the cornea.

Since the largest cornea may be 13.00 mm. in diameter, most corneal lenses are smaller than this.

When made of hard material the lenses can be as small as 6.5 mm. in diameter and as thin as 0.10 mm. When made of softer materials they can vary in size up to 12.50 mm. in size, and 0.15 to 0.30 mm. thick, depending upon the material and power.

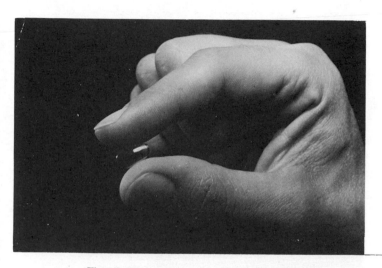

Fig. 19 Soft lens being flexed (B. & L. Soflens).

Materials used for Corneal and Corneo-scleral Lenses:

PMMA (Perspex)	1.4% water content
P.HEMA (hydrophilic)	40% water content
P.HEMA Co-polymers (hydrophilic)	40% to 70% water content
Vinyl Acrylate Co-polymers (hydrophilic)	3% to 85% water content
Silicon Rubber	No water

If PMMA is used several tints are possible, and a limited number with soft materials.

Special Corneal Lenses

In order to fit the cornea accurately, the harder lens has been made with a choice of several back surfaces:

    e.g. Multispherical
        True conoid
        Pseudo Conoidal — Offset Curves
                         — Tangent Surfaces

Non-Round Lenses

The lens is made △ or ▭ to prevent rotation. The use of small depressions, holes or elevations on the back of the lens does the same thing.

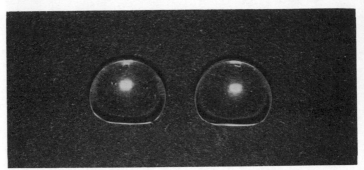

Fig. 20 Special type Corneal Lens to correct astigmatism.

Prism Lenses

The lens is made thicker below, so that it will settle on the eye always in one position. This is done so that either more than one vision (bifocals) can be ground onto the lens, or if cylindrical powers are required to correct residual astigmatism. Soft lenses can also be made in this form.

Holes in Lenses

They are often useful to allow better respiration of the surface of the cornea. This may cure fogging of vision common after several hours of wear.

Chapter VI

THE FITTING OF THE CONTACT LENS

At the first or second consultation the patient has certain routine measurements done on the eye and vision. These measurements may be, in themselves, extensive if there is any evidence of abnormality. In the normal eye with a low error of refraction the tests are usually confined to testing of sight and the correction by spectacle trial lenses; colour vision tests if not done before; the measurement of the field of vision; the examination of the front surface of the eye and lids using a special microscope, the measurement of the front curvature of the cornea; the diameter of the cornea, which is about 1 mm. larger than the coloured (iris) part of the eye and the diameter of the pupil. All these measurements will be used to formulate the prescription of the contact lens.

It is important at this time to describe the fitting rationale that the contact lens practitioner follows. The first principle is to use as little material as possible consistent with keeping the lens on the eye and centred over the cornea. These are optical necessities concerned with obtaining good vision. For the sake of comfort the lens must fit the eye without undue rubbing or scratching in all positions of gaze and with all types of blinking of the lids. Essentially a lens that adheres to the eye and moves with the eye is comfortable. If this type of glove-like fit can be worn without pressure on the eye at any one point or area then well and good. If, furthermore, the glove-like fit permits free flow of air and tears to the eye and waste products to leave the eye's surface then better still. Even with all the materials available: some with good moulding properties, others rigid; some with good air flow, others bad, the final functional lens is a compromise. The eye and lids will have to adapt to the abnormal sensation, the vision will not be natural or the same as spectacle vision. The eye will have to survive and compensate with different pressures

of gases, different concentrations of enzymes and other important organic chemicals. This takes time and adaptation to a contact
lens may be impossible for some very sensitive individuals or
where the eye power, shape, or health is abnormal.

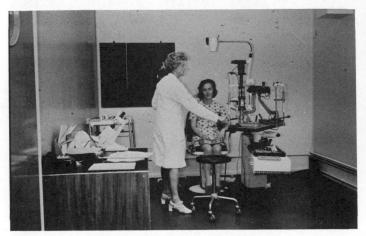

Fig. 21 Combined Diagnostic Unit.

The eye can be fitted entirely upon mathematical formulae.
Given that the radius of curvature of the cornea at the centre
is a given number of millimetres, it is possible to determine the
back surface of the contact lens. For hard materials the back
surface of the contact lens must overall be very slightly flatter
than the front surface of the eye. This will permit some movement of the lens. This slight movement allows tear fluid to pass
both in front of the lens and behind. The flow of fluid brings
air to the front of the eye and allows normal respiration. If the
material is not rigid it will tend to mould to the eye curves. The
fitter must decide how much of a moulded fit is permissible. With
very soft materials and good air flow through the material a complete glove fit is permissible. One may well ask why not fit everyone with the same material. If soft materials containing a lot of
water give the greatest comfort, then fit everyone with such
lenses. The answer is that best vision cannot always be obtained
with soft lenses. This is especially true if the eye has an irregular

shape. It may be possible to determine which particular material to use to give the best vision and comfort. It will be confusing to the reader to speak of so many materials. Therefore the two extremes will be taken. —Hard plastic materials and how they are fitted and soft lenses at the other end of the scale. The comparison of the extremes will help orientate the uninitiated.

Fitting

By making lenses very thin (0.1 mm. or less) it is possible with just one back curve and an edge back curve to fit just the spherical centre of the cornea. This area varies from 5.50 to 8.50 mm. in diameter. Providing the powers required are low, this is possible. In practice, it is necessary to have lenses at least 6.5 mm. in diameter, otherwise a good image is not formed. Using this principle, all such lenses would vary from 6.5 to 9.0 in size. Whilst it is possible to measure the diameter of the central spherical zone of the cornea it is not necessary. We know that the large head has the large eye with the flatter curvature, and vice versa the small head the small eye and steep curved cornea. Therefore it is easy to relate the curvature, which can be easily measured with a keratometer* to the diameter. Thus a steep corneal centre reading of 7.00 mm. requires a diameter of 7 and a flat curvature of 8.50 a diameter of 8.50. In practice, most hard lens fittings are between 7.50 and 9.00 when based upon this understanding. If for any reason a large lens has to be used for a small eye with steep curvatures, then one or more peripheral curves must be used, so that the outer and flatter surfaces of the cornea are fitted correctly.

  The practitioner will explain to the patient that there are two main points for discussion which may involve the patient in a choice. The soft materials will be more comfortable in the first few hours of wear. Acceptance of the lens can in some patients be almost immediately. As the period of wear increases some discomfort can occur. This discomfort will depend upon how much the lens occludes the cornea from air and tear fluid. It will also depend upon how well the lens fits the eye. In some instances and for special sized lenses permanent wear for several days' trial wear may be advised, but in most cases a gradual

* *Keratometer = instrument for measuring corneal curvatures.*

increase from, say, 6 hours to 15 hours daily is the more usual pattern. More will be said about the permanently worn lens later. With soft lenses, providing there is no large degree of astigmatism or corneal irregularity, almost normal vision can be expected. The vision may appear to have a slight water or grease haze if the tears are abnormal. This type of vision is acceptable to 95% of the contact lens wearing population but not by all. Some individuals are very sensitive to any defect in clear vision. The practitioner will explain that softer materials are more expensive to maintain, since they cannot last as long as hard. Depending upon the care taken and the quality of the patient's tears, soft lenses can last as long as 3 years. On the other hand, some patients repeatedly break lenses even after a few days' use. These problems of management will be discussed in the next chapter.

The practitioner will then describe the corneal or scleral hard lens. In normal eye curvatures it may be the small corneal lens that will be fitted. The patient will be told that even 3 months may be necessary to completely accept the lens; that if a small thin design is used the majority can wear all day after a few days' gradual build-up; that in some instances all day wear can be achieved immediately. But some discomfort is common. Dust and wind can be troublesome with this type of lens and it may fall off the eye.

The fitting, as stated, can be done entirely from measurement. This is also true for most soft lens designs and for small hard lenses, but for in-between sizes where the peripheral cornea has to play a part in centring and stabilising the lens, the use of trial lenses is necessary. Therefore most practitioners have sets of trial lenses, both hard and soft. Some even have large stocks of lenses, so that most common powers and fittings can be issued from stock. It must be appreciated that with increments in power of $\frac{1}{4}$ of a unit (dioptre) and variations in power from +20.00 to −20.00, together with different combinations of size and curvatures, millions of variations are possible. This is not even including variations in material and thickness. But for common powers between +4.00 to −8.00 and especially with soft materials, where there is only a small range of fitting variations, lenses from stock are possible.

One may therefore ask why aren't all soft lenses issued from stock? The answer is that if a soft lens can be reproduced exactly to a prescription and ordered from a trial lens fitting, then there is no need to keep a stock of lenses. But where lenses are not exactly reproduceable, then it is best to issue a lens from stock. To hold large stocks of perishable, damageable lenses is inadvisable, both for patient and practitioner.

Many practitioners like to use trial or diagnostic lenses, so that the patient obtains some idea of what the initial sensation will be. Furthermore, with additional spectacle trial lenses, the patient can be told and shown how normal the vision will be. By the trial lens method problems of astigmatism that cannot be corrected by the contact lens can best be evaluated.

If the practitioner does not use a trial lens technique, there is no cause for alarm. Some practitioners prefer to order a lens that mathematically may be one hundred per cent the correct lens. If it is not, then it can be altered or changed for one that is. This two-stage fitting using a newly manufactured lens is more expensive to the practitioner than the trial lens technique and has much to commend it. Trial lenses, themselves, can be suspect. They may be old and wearing out, incorrect because of age and not the best comfort because of material and design.

The assessment of the fit is a combination of several factors. The patient must wear the soft lens for at least 15 minutes to 1 hour before the vision is checked. The sensation of large lenses is felt usually by the lower lid and this becomes less after a few hours. For small hard lenses the eye may become red and sore. The lids can swell and tears do not stop. Normal blinking is difficult but must be achieved if successful wear is to be won. The practitioner will examine the position of the lens and the eyes' reaction to the lens by magnification methods, including the microscope. The use of a fluorescent dye is possible with some lens materials. This gives the practitioner a good idea of where tears are flowing or are held by the lens. It is necessary to view the eye with blue light to obtain best fluorescence. Only a mere drop of fluorescine producing concentrations of 10^{-6} (1 in 10,000,000 pts.) being necessary. Thus if the lens fits too steeply the dye will concentrate behind the lens at the centre. On the other hand, if it fits flatly, then the concentration will be towards the periphery.

If the cornea touches the lens no fluorescence will be present at the zones of contact. A good edge to a lens will not dig into the tissue and the presence of a thin band of dye around the edge will show this. The same dye will also show whether the eye tissues are damaged in any way at the surface. Even minute abrasions unbeknown to exist by the patient and of no significance can be examined by the use of this fluorescent dye.

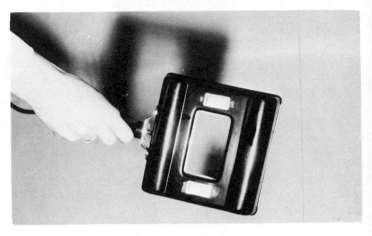

Fig. 22a Blue light.

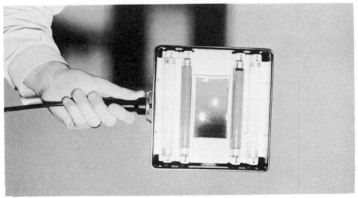

Fig. 22b Blue light.

Gross errors in power and fit are not allowed by the practitioner, but it is often expedient to allow small errors to remain until some tolerance to wear has been proven. The period of adaptation is important, both to the patient and practitioner.

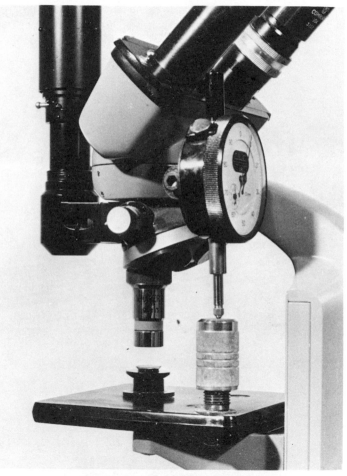

Fig. 23 Checking the curves of a lens.
Radiuscope (photo by Smith & Nephew Ltd.)

Unless the patient has trust and faith in the practitioner, they will tend to interpret their failure to tolerate a lens as practitioner incompetence this may rarely be the true cause of intolerance for the average wearer. The practitioner knows that the eye and lens can undergo changes in the first few weeks of wear. The eye, itself, may swell very slightly, enough to change the fitting pattern. The lens may also change its curves and power, sometimes the combination of both leads to discomfort and poor vision. It is then a problem. If

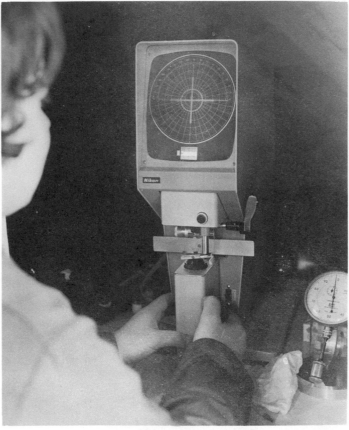

Fig. 24 Focimeter to check the powers.

the patient's eye adapts to the lens and returns to its normal power and curvatures, then the lens may still be wrong but can be corrected. If the practitioner changes the lens to accommodate the eye, the final result may be a bad fit. It is a period, therefore, where the patient must have patience but should not last longer than 3 months for any type of lens except where progressive disease of the eye is present. The correction of the problems that can arise after wear has commenced and necessitating alteration or changes in lens design or material will be described in the next chapter.

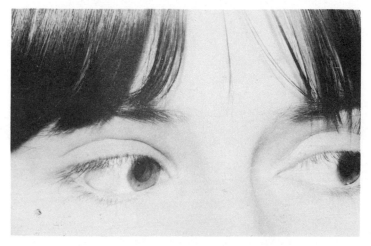

Fig. 25 Normal eye with myopia fitted with soft lens.

The practitioner or assistant will, after making sure that the best vision and fitting are available, begin to instruct the patient. The instruction is best on a person to person basis. Films, pictures and booklets are good adjuncts but cannot replace a one to one relationship with the instructor.

All lenses must be inserted wet. It is most important that the correct solution be used. If in doubt, fresh normal saline without preservative can be used: boiling pure water with cooking salt for 10 minutes. One pint of water to 1 level teaspoon of salt will give the correct physiological concentration. Salt tablets bought from the chemist and pure water will make the best solution. The latter can be used for soft lenses. Commercial preparations are available. They should state which type of lens they are to be used for.

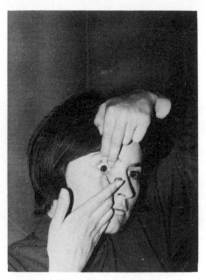

Fig. 26 To show method of inserting and removing a hard corneal lens. *N.B.* Misplaced lenses can either be removed or gently massaged back onto the eye.

For low water content lenses, that is the conventional hard material lens, most solutions on the market containing wetting agents, cleaning agents, disinfecting chemicals are usable, but on *no* account must such single purpose or combined solutions be used on soft wet lenses. The reason for this is that the chemicals become selectively absorbed and can cause deterioration of the plastic and often pain or even damage to the eye surface. There are specially prepared solutions, mostly containing organic mercury as a preservative and germicide, together with other physiological salts to provide a solution which is stabile and very similar to tears. These solutions can be used to store wet lenses but must not be boiled. Upon boiling such solutions the salts may become con-

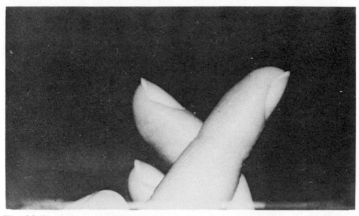

Fig. 27 To show method of inserting and removing a hard corneal lens. *N.B.* Misplaced lenses can either be removed or gently massaged back onto the eye.

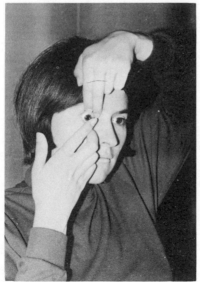

Fig. 28 To show method of inserting and removing a hard corneal lens. *N.B.* Misplaced lenses can either be removed or gently massaged back onto the eye.

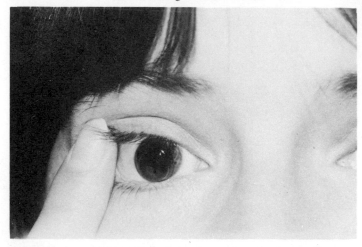

Fig. 29 To show method of inserting and removing a hard corneal lens. *N.B.* Misplaced lenses can either be removed or gently massaged back onto the eye.

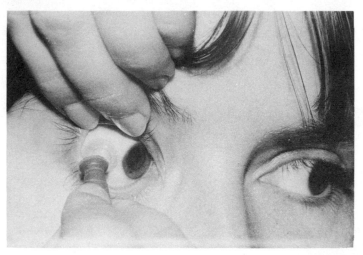

Fig. 30 To show method of inserting and removing a hard corneal lens. *N.B.* Misplaced lenses can either be removed or gently massaged back onto the eye.

centrated and precipitate out of solution and spoil the lens. Therefore, at present, the only solution that can be safely used by the
patient for heating soft wet lenses is *N* saline.

It is not uncommon for each practitioner to recommend cleaning agents for lenses. They must be washed off the lens before
use. For hard lenses such cleaning agents have included paraffin,
metal polish and vinegar! For soft lenses medical protein dissolv-
ing agents and enzymes able to dissolve proteins have been used.

The patient learns how to store the lens in the special container, then how to remove the lens without causing damage. Next
how to hold the lens on the middle or index finger and for bigger

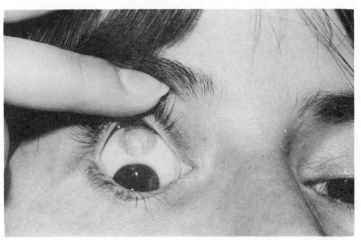

Fig. 31 To show method of inserting and removing a hard corneal lens.
N.B. Misplaced lenses can either be removed or gently massaged back onto
the eye.

lenses in the tripod formed by holding thumb, first and second
finger tips together. The other hand holds the upper lid up. The
same hand can also spare a finger to depress the lower lid. The
lens is then placed on the eye. Often the aim is incorrect and the
lens lands on the white of the eye. Providing the eye has tears, it
is possible to gently massage the lens back onto cornea through
the lid or with a mirror to gently lead the lens with the smallest
finger tip back to the centre.

Very large scleral lenses have to be filled with fluid, the head bent down and the lens, which is held horizontal, slipped and held under the upper lid but against the eye. The large lens can be removed by placing the finger on the upper edge and elevating the upper lid at the same time. The downward movement of the eye will then result in the lens coming out of the eye.

The small hard lenses can be removed by placing a sucker on the lens and tilting, or by tightening the lids outwards and upwards. A slight downward movement of the eye will express the lens. Soft lenses can be removed by touching the front of the lens and moving it downwards. The eye looks up and, whilst the finger steadies the lens which is now on the white of the eye, a gentle pinching movement will remove the lens from the eye. Alternatively, the lens can be removed by gently squeezing the upper and lower lid together but with an action (scissor like) that is away from each other. The lens will then be squeezed from the eye. This method can also be used for hard small lenses. Every patient must with the help of the teacher discover which method will produce the best results without hurting the eye or lens. No sudden or rough movements are permissible.

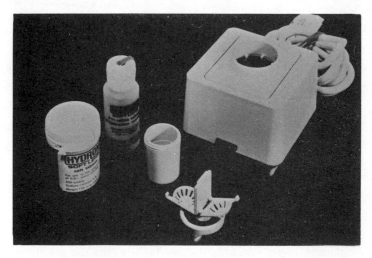

Fig. 32 Disinfection kit for soft (Hydron) lenses. N.B. Electric boiler.

Once the patient has mastered the insertion and removal technique and the use of solution lubrication drops or any other treatments advised the wearing pattern time-table begins. To try and wear contact lenses other than constant wear at the end or beginning of a busy day requiring critical vision is not fair on the eye or the lens. It is best to start over a weekend. Once they are in, activities requiring non-critical use of the eyes are advised. Walking in the open is the best way to commence. When one returns it is wise to avoid hot dry atmospheres. Initially rapid blinking is essential to keep the lenses moist and the vision at its best. The lenses should not be interchanged unless they are exactly the same. It is often wise to ensure that even identical lenses are marked with different code letters or symbols.

The practitioner will change or modify the lenses at follow-up visits. Whilst hard lenses can be modified in size and curvature very slightly and power also altered by 0.75 of a unit (dioptre), it is difficult to alter a soft lens. Such lenses, if unsatisfactory, have to be exchanged. It is important for the practitioner to see the patient frequently in the first few weeks if there are complications.

Scleral Lenses (Hard)

These lenses are made from a model eye prepared in plaster from a "gel" impression taken of the front of the eye. The lens is modified to fit the eye and finally the power required is added to the front optic (centre) portion. This process may take several visits, and requires the services of a skilled practitioner (see page 35).

Chapter VII

COMPLICATIONS

The reasons why patients fail to wear contact lenses are as important as the fitting. The eye was not designed or developed biologically to wear a plastic membrane, such as the contact lens. Therefore it is always a question of can an individual adapt to the appliance. Adaptation occurs at several levels. There is the sensory adaptation to the lens. The presence of a smooth shell or lens on the eye is something of a shock in the first instance. Depending upon the psychological background of the individual, the severity of the shock can vary. There are some who can touch their own eye without inhibitions but there are others who have a taboo about the eyes. The latter individuals cannot stand the thought, let alone the presence, of a foreign body (even drops) entering the eye. Previous experience of pain in the eye from a sharp piece of grit or dust may be the underlying cause. In some instances the personality of the individual is so sensitive that contact lenses could only be inserted under hypnosis or some form of anaesthesia. Such patients should not have contact lenses unless their basic personality disorder has medical treatment. Nevertheless, even very sensitive persons have persevered and exerted their will to overcome the fear of wearing a contact lens. The desire to appear normal is overwhelmingly strong in some persons and sufficient to overcome abnormal sensitivity. To such persons spectacles, irrespective of their design, do not enhance their appearance.

The sensation of pain is protective against injury and once the lens has been inserted and, providing it is of optimum minimal thickness and a good fit, the eye and lids will accept the sensation. The adaptation to a smooth plastic conforming shape placed on the eye and decrease of pain sensation may only be a matter of ten to twenty minutes. The initial discomfort phase is associated with lacrimation, which can be quite troublesome. Very sensitive persons also reflexly close the eyes in a spasm. This will increase the pain, especially if the lenses are a poor fit or in the wrong position. Congestion of the lids with swelling occurs from such lid closure spasms and the eye is often very red. Unless the spasm ceases and is replaced by relaxed blinking, there is little hope for success.

Sensitivity may be at a higher level of the nervous system. Thus the whole body may react to the procedure of insertion of the lens. As the lids are touched by the practitioner or even at the sight of the lens, the patient may attempt quite violently to withdraw. They may attempt to climb out of the chair, arch their back and tensely tighten every stretch muscle in their body. It is quite useless to proceed with the procedure of insertion. The patient requires a long time to be spent in explaining and analysing the cause of the fear. It is best such patients see another patient using lenses and then after instruction let the patient place their lens in the eye. Surprisingly enough, a high percentage of sensitive individuals can manage to handle the lens and insert it without the help of another person. These forms of sensitivity are chiefly reflex nerve actions and often beyond the control of the patient, but they do persist even after the patient has success-fully worn lenses for several years. 1 in 20 patients feels faint or does completely faint after the lens or a drop has been placed in the eye. There is also a reflex action of eye sensation affecting the heart. People who faint more than twice with contact lens insertion should be warned not to proceed unless they have seen a physician and had the go ahead from him.

For the normal person the initial discomfort is followed by a period of relative ease. Then after about an hour a warm feeling is experienced over one or more parts of the eye. This indicates that the lens has caused some white part of the eye to become inflamed. With very small thin hard or soft large lenses this may not occur. The awareness of the lens by the lids can result in irritation and often a gritty sensation, but this is often a late response. Some patients say that the eyes feel cold with contact lens wear. This may be due to abnormal blinking and rapid evaporation of tears from the eye surface. When the lens is worn outdoors dust may enter the eye and become lodged either under the lid or lens. This can cause acute pain and reflex lacrimation, the latter being sufficient in most instances to wash the dust away. Older patients sometimes do not have the abundance of tear secretion necessary for successful wear. It soon becomes obvious that tears, the essential lubricant for good wear, are deficient and contact lens tolerance will be limited. The younger successful wearer will also notice tear drying problems. Dry rapid moving air can be encountered in ventilating systems, in sports (skiing and driving). Rapid drying of the eye results in a lens adhering to the eye tissue and causing either pain or lifting of the lens off the eye and its loss, or both.

It is as well to discuss the environment in association with contact lens wear. The ideal atmosphere for contact lens wear is a cool, windless day with normal humidity. The air should be unpolluted. Unfortunately this is rarely obtainable. The atmosphere of the home, office and factory can be polluted with irritating smoke, chemical fumes, cement and building dust, pollens and so forth. Even persons not wearing contact lenses are affected by the atmosphere in contact with their eyes. Therefore it is often much worse when wearing a contact lens. On the other hand, the area of cornea in contact with the lens is protected. Thus there is increasing evidence if splashes of chemicals into the eyes occur or injury to the eye, the lens will protect the cornea. However, if the remainder of the eye is affected by the injury, the contact lens may still prove to be a complicating factor. A good example of this is flash welding. The flash has a very high intensity of ultra-violet light. This causes a burn of the eye tissues. If protective goggles are not worn, the eye burns, especially on the exposed portions of the cornea, can become severely inconvenienced by the contact lens, even though the cornea under the lens is unaffected. Work at furnaces or where infra-red light is emitted will also cause burns of the eye, and protective glasses must be worn.

Some patients are allergic or sensitive to many things. It could be the pollen of flowers or grass, the dust of the carpet, the hairs of animals and so on. Many individuals are sensitive to drugs, even simple drugs, such as aspirin or the preservatives used in eye drop lotions and contact lens solutions.

Some patients do give a history of such problems and this is helpful, but others may not have symptoms until after commencing contact lens wear. It is often difficult without tests to determine whether the eye is showing an allergic reaction or just an irritation or infection. The use of anti-allergic drugs as eye drops or even tablets by mouth can help. It is often necessary to decrease or even stop contact lens wear during an allergic attack. Needless to say, the causative agent, if known, must be avoided.

Many patients have skin disorders that are indicative of sensitive skins. They are often associated with similar problems affecting the lids or even the eye. The use of contact lenses in such sufferers must be problematical.

As previously stated, insufficient tears or abnormal tears will cause problems for the contact lens wearer. The association of rheumatism anaemia with dryness of the eyes may not be generally known, but often such patients may give a story of gritty sensation and dry feeling of the eyes, even before contact lenses were worn. If conventional small hard lenses are worn, they are likely to fail. The only type that can be worn with comfort are very soft lenses and then only minimally. There is some connection between tears and the health of the front of the eye. If the tears are abnormal, the epithelium (see page 10) will show signs of minute erosions. They can only be seen in detail with magnification of x10 to x40. They can occur from rubbing the cornea or spontaneously from death of the small cells. We think that abnormal tears and contact lens wear will cause this to happen. We know that lack of oxygen will also result in similar changes, often precursed by swelling of the cells. Pregnancy, certain times in the menstrual period and taking the pill will in about 1 in 10 women make them more sensitive to these changes. When they are severe contact lens wearing becomes difficult. One patient affected by this problem said 'The only time I want to wear contact lenses is when I am on the pill'. Certainly there is less need to wear contact lenses for appearance during late pregnancy. Therefore the paradox of wanting contact lenses to attract the male species but being unable to maintain wear is frustrating.

The great danger with all contact lenses is the development of corneal ulcers. There is a great deal of misunderstanding amongst the public regarding ulcers of the eye. Some persons who have little white or clear cysts along the eye margin think they have ulcers. But, in fact, they are no more than signs of excessive gland function and easily treatable and of little significance. Others evert the lids and see small white concretions in the skin of the inner lid and they also think they have ulcers. They are not ulcers but only a predilection for chalky or fatty deposits to collect. The same deposits can occur on either side of the cornea between the lids. It is of little significance and after diagnosis may not be treated. The upper lid inside and towards the nose is often red, even in normal eyes, and slightly elevated if the upper lid is everted. Again, it is of little significance. True ulcers of the front of the eye are very rare, very painful and associated with loss of vision. It is rarely a complication of normal eye contact lens wear, but can occur in diseased eyes wearing contact lenses.

Overwear of contact lenses is the commonest cause of trouble. Hard lenses can be worn comfortably once the front of the eye and lid are adapted to the sensation, but it is significant that this is associated with some loss of sensation of the eye tissue. Thus a vicious circle can occur in some patients. The lens may be a cause of trauma to the eye but the longer it is worn the more comfortable the eye is. Alas, when the trauma is excessive and the lens is removed then the eye becomes acutely painful and often requires treatment. Alternatively, the eye begins to reject the lens by a very slow process. The patient realises that every day the comfort is decreasing. When the all-day wearer can only tolerate 8 hours they seek advice. The cause of rejection is not completely known. It may be allergy to the eye's own cells, which are constantly being traumatised (however minutely) by contact lens wear. The nerves of the eye associated with pain sensation may have become suddenly more sensitive or the chemicals and hormones that determine their function changed. Causes such as change of environment, drugs or wearing out of the lens are suspect but rarely proven. Eye discomfort and pain after achieving good tolerance with the contact lens is an enigma. But one thing is certain, the perfect contact lens does not cause such problems. It has yet to be invented and, when it does arrive, research will have to prove that the lens does work physiologically with the normal eye. This applies especially to constant wear soft lenses.

Redness of the eye is a reflex protective phenomenon. Thus

the diseased or injured eye has dilatation of its blood vessels, more blood being necessary to fight infection and heal tissues. For contact lens wearers it is only the lids and white part of the eye that become red. Rarely the transparent cornea can develop new blood vessels. This is, of course, a serious complication if it occurs towards the centre of the sight. But the vessels are often so

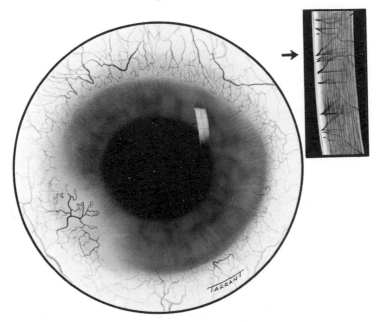

Fig. 33 To show blood vessels and scarring of cornea due to prolonged wear of hard scleral lens.
(Reproduced by permission of Mr. T. Tarrant)

minute that only a microscope and a skilled practitioner will be able to diagnose their presence. As stated for disease, blood vessels will bring increased nutrients and systems for fighting infection. Therefore their presence is advantageous. Their persistence, however, can lead to deterioration of vision when present in transparent tissues. Their constant presence on the white of the eye will lead to an unsightly appearance. The earlier in life they appear and the longer they stay the more difficult it is to make them disappear, even with treatment. Whenever the eye becomes red, especially if associated with pain and/or loss of clear vision, a medical opinion must be sought without too much delay.

In contact lens wear there can be several causes of red eyes. — From the very simple things like bruising of the eye due to poor contact lens insertion and removal to more serious problems such as infection. It is important for the practitioner to establish the cause and eliminate the problem. It may require even a change of lens material.

Infection is a dreaded complication for the contact lens wearer, but, in fact, serious infection occurs only rarely and need not worry the patient. There are certain basic principles that must be known. The lens, if stored in a solution — and this applies to many contact lenses must only be stored in a solution sterile at the time of purchase. Once the container is opened, then infection of the contents can occur. Unless this simple rule is followed the manufacturer, practitioner and patient could all infect the lens. Therefore if a solution does not contain germicides and preservatives, it must be disinfected by heating with the lens (see pages 49, 50, 53). This remark is especially true for all soft lenses containing a high quantity of water. An infected lens does not necessarily mean an infected eye. It does mean for soft lenses a spoilt lens. Hard lenses require different solutions. They may even be stored dry but must be inserted wet. Most solutions which do not require heat sterilization contain preservatives, but they are weak preservatives and therefore sufficient time and quantity of fluid is necessary to bathe the lens in order to get rid of germs. If the patient is sensitive to a particular germ, then infection can occur, but rarely otherwise.

Infection is nearly always associated with swelling, redness, pain of the eye and also a discharge. This discharge can be coloured white or yellow. Contact lens wear must be stopped and treatment obtained. It is important to know that the habits of some humans are far from clean. Therefore the use of contact lenses presents another hazard in their lives. Furthermore, many individuals are susceptible to eye infection and, once again, the contact lens may be unjustly accused of causing eye infection.

If the contact lens irritates the portion under the upper lid, then a swelling of the lid can occur and the lid will appear slightly lower than normal. Treatment combined with alterations in the lens may be necessary. In some countries where trachoma is prevalent the patient may be more prone to these inflammatory reactions and they can also involve the cornea. Therefore if there has been, or even suspected, eye disease, a consultation with an ophthalmologist is necessary.

Since contact lens wear is often associated with lid discomfort many patients try to avoid blinking. They may stare, blink abnormally, or hold the lids very tight. These lid postures are abnormal and must be avoided. Frequent and relaxed closure of the lids is essential for good contact lens wear. Unless the front of the eye and lens are kept wet with a tear film good vision and comfort are not possible.

Optical

Gradual clouding of vision with streaks of light radiating from isolated lights or even coloured haloes indicate that the front of the eye is starved of oxygen. Unless the oxygen can be obtained from the eye itself or the tissues compensate for this deficiency, the skin of the cornea will become swollen and show evidence of microscopic degeneration of the individual cells. Before that can happen the eye often becomes painful and the sight worse. But there are rare examples of patients sleeping with hard contact lenses without problems. On the other hand, the complications can be severe. In most instances they are reversible problems. All contact lens wearers experience these problems in a minor way, especially during the first few months of wear. This is especially noticeable in some patients who wear soft contact lenses constantly night and day. In these patients the swelling of the cornea and the clouding of vision occurs upon wakening in the morning and disappears later in the day.

Some patients may never achieve tolerance for all day wear, irrespective of the lens worn. When they revert to spectacles the vision can be blurred. Habitual hard lens wearers may find that this blurring lasts for several days, even weeks. The majority find that after a few hours the spectacle acuity is satisfactory. Patients who wear hard lenses only a few hours daily will not have this problem, and it also does not affect soft lens wearers.

The cause is in part oedema of the cornea but also distortion of the corneal curvature. Only rarely does the distortion become persistent and does not affect sight more than 10% except in rare instances. Small thin hard corneal lenses cause less distortion after daily wear than large thick lenses.

The contact lens will correct vision. It has its own optical imperfections that some individuals cannot tolerate. Whilst the practitioner may consider such patients, who may even see the bottom line of the chart, as fastidious or peculiar, they are being truthful.

The contact lens that is too mobile will only intermittently give good vision. It will also introduce a prism* effect as the lens moves across the line of sight. Spectacles give a constant prism effect for each eye. The effect varies as we look away from the centre of the lens but the degree is always constant and this also applies for both eyes. With good fitting and good wearing the lens will centre over the line of sight most of the time and most patients do not suffer from the problems of image movement. If this problem cannot be solved by larger or different lens design, then contact lens wear may have to be abandoned.

The other optical defects are multi-image formation, glare from the edge and watery haze due to tears. The effects of mucous and lid secretions can cause hazy images. Some of these defects cannot be solved and contact lens wear may have to be abandoned.

In short-sighted individuals the better panoramic vision and larger image may be a bonus for distance vision but the reverse is true for near. They often complain that reading is difficult. The small lenses may decentre when the eyes converge and near sight becomes difficult. For individuals over forty the focusing becomes difficult until at 60 it may be lost completely. The wearing of contact lenses accentuates this problem. It can be solved in several ways. One easy way is to under-correct the distance myopic vision and ensure that the lens size and fitting gives a good optical result. The other is to undercorrect the eye that is non-dominant, thus leaving the dominant eye for distance vision and the other for near correction. It is also possible to order spectacles to be worn for reading. Bifocal spectacles can also be worn occasionally for reading.

*prism = optical displacement of the image.

Bifocal contact lenses are possible for hard and soft lenses but do not work for everyone. Much depends upon the power, size of lens and fitting whether a bifocal contact lens will work. If the patient is willing to face the expense of several trial contact lenses, then they can be tried.

Double vision, due to weakness of binocular vision, is not uncommon. Young persons may compensate but older patients may have to give up contact lens wear. Such weaknesses in some patients are best treated by spectacles which have either a beneficial prism element or prism power can be introduced into the spectacle lens. With contact lenses the power may be correct but the prism effect can be the opposite of that required. Therefore when this occurs the two eyes cannot easily work together and sometimes double vision results.

One must realise that, providing the patient and practitioner work as a team to achieve the best result, most problems can be overcome. But in some instances after expenditure of professional time and many lenses failure is the end result. Neither the patient or practitioner is to blame and any individual who enters upon contact lens fitting without realising that some expense is involved whether they are successful or not is foolish in the extreme. On the other hand, for a practitioner to over commercialise contact lenses by reducing the professional time costs to zero must be condemned as bad practice and not in the patient's interest, the inference being that in the difficult case he is unlikely to wish to spend any time other than the minimum.

Chapter VIII

THE USE OF CONTACT LENSES FOR TREATMENT OF EYE DISEASE—INCLUDING DIAGNOSIS, EXPERIMENTAL AND PROSTHETICS (ARTIFICIAL EYES)

The preceding chapters have dealt with the correction of normal errors of eye power, but there are many causes of power abnormalities that are caused by old or still active disease. In some instances, the disease is quiescent or has been surgically treated and in others the use of the contact lens is necessary in the presence of active disease. Whilst the majority of instances require the lens to correct sight, there are others where the lens has a different function.

The lens may be required to function as a mechanical barrier. For very thin soft lenses this barrier can indeed be thought of as a membrane. Such a membrane separating the front of the eye from the lids and atmosphere may be called by some practitioners a protective or bandage lens. The power of the lens may be immaterial since the function is not to give vision. In many such instances the eye may be beyond good sight.

Apart from the protective function, there are drug dispensation techniques. It is possible either to charge the lens with drugs (e.g. hydrophilic lenses and water soluble drugs) or place the drug solutions or ointments in the lens itself.

There is no end to the ideas and application of contact lenses for different eye diseases and it would be best to describe a few common eye diseases and outline the special contact lens treatments applied.

Abnormal Eye Powers

Very high degrees of short-sight or long-sight require thick spectacle lenses. The power is often reduced to a small area of the lens, so as to reduce the weight and aberrations of the lenses. If the patient can tolerate contact lenses, then a better form of correction is possible. For example, in short-sight not only would the contact lens increase the size of the image and therefore permit improved vision but also allow a much larger field of vision to be corrected and allow the eyes to move from side to side without the visual restrictions of the thick edges of high power spectacles. Several infections and degenerations of the cornea result in scarring which results in abnormal curvatures. It is not unusual for such curvatures to be uncorrectable by spectacles and contact lenses will negate the effect of the scar tissue and, in some instances, give almost normal sight.

Keratoconus (Conical Cornea)

A good example of abnormal curvature associated with scarring and thinning of the front of the eye is keratoconus. It affects possibly one in ten thousand persons and appears to have some inherited and environmental factors. It is a condition that has a slow onset in infancy and accelerates in puberty. Most individuals affected have one weak eye and may end up with both affected. By middle age most patients have become compensated. But at least ten per cent. may need a graft operation in one eye to obtain good vision. Since the success rate of this operation in good hands is as high as 90% the outcome is usually good. This particular abnormality of the cornea can be corrected by the contact lens and result in good vision. Unfortunately 50% of these patients cannot tolerate contact lenses all day. Soft lenses do not always give the best vision. Combinations of hard and soft lenses are sometimes tried. The good practitioner may have to try all types of lenses. If no contact lens can be worn and the vision is poor, then operation is often advised. Patients will often seek out new and bizarre treatments for this condition and it is advisable that such treatments should only be tried if an ophthalmic surgeon is agreeable. Even after successful graft surgery, the eye may have to be fitted with a contact lens to obtain good vision. In at least 50% of patients good vision is even obtainable with spectacle lenses. Thus a successful outcome may mean the restoration of good sight where previously registrable blindness was present.

Aphakia

The medical term means an eye without an internal lens. The lens has been lost, displaced or removed. It is commonly the condition of an eye treated for cataract, cataract being the clouding over of the clear internal lens of the eye. If this powerful lens is damaged or removed, then the eye becomes a much weaker power. In order to see clearly, the eye must have placed in front of it a high power plus lens like a magnifying lens to condense the rays of light in the same way as the human lens. Unfortunately such a correction worn as spectacles is not always tolerated. The patient may complain of objects looking larger than normal. Also the area over which one can see is severely restricted. If only one eye is aphakic, then it is often impossible for the two eyes which see differently to again work together. The aphakic eye corrected by a contact lens is almost optically normal and many of the original problems disappear. All types of lenses can be used for this condition and some patients are able to wear some forms of softer materials constantly. The future, therefore, looks even better for patients who have to have their cataracts removed.

Albinos

Patients born without pigment will have poor vision and sometimes shaky eyes (nystagmus). Their appearance can be improved by wearing tinted or coloured contact lenses. If they have a high power abnormality, their vision may also be marginally improved. But it is wrong to hold out too much hope for the improvement of this problem. One sincerely hopes that the missing hormone and metabolic error will eventually be treated by medical methods and not the contact lens.

Disfigured and Abnormal Eyes

To mask defects partially or completely the contact lens can be made of coloured material or paints used on its surface. Thus the whole eye can be made to look normal. If vision is required, then the centre pupil can be left clear and with an optical power. Some children are born with one eye not developed or early infection can produce the same result. The eye will appear small and sunken as the face grows. It is often possible, but not always, to fit a coloured shell to the abnormal side and make the patient look almost 100% normal. It is never possible using plastics and the cleverest colouring to simulate complete normality, but one must remember that we only rarely look at another's eyes at very close range and many people with such appliances pass for normal.

Absent Eyes

Some eyes have to be removed, for example, following severe injuries and disease. The surgeon will often be able to replace the eye with a plastic globe. This implant is much smaller than a normal eye. The eye muscles can even be attached to the implant. In some instances the outer eye surface can be retained but the interior of the eye filled with a plastic globe. The final shell fitted may have to be thick or thin but is moulded to the space left behind. It is painted and covered with plastic to simulate a normal eye. Even red nylon thread is added to give the appearance of blood vessels. The results are extremely good and movement of the artificial appliance can almost give the appearance of normality. Very often the tissues around the eye may appear abnormal but can rarely be treated. Unfortunately some individuals quite understandably make an obsession about the loss of an eye and will worry to the extent of causing mental illness if absolute perfection is not possible.

Dry Eyes

Many eyes become blind due to abnormal tears or absence of tears. The original cause may have been severe infections of the eyes or general diseases, such as rheumatism, that are associated with loss of normal tear formation.

Not all eyes can be helped by a protective contact lens. Since the basic condition is desperate, the treatment may be advised. Unfortunately the outcome may not be happy. Rarely contact lenses can be a cause of recurrent problems themselves. The medical specialist must try to assess whether the good points outweigh the complications. Since many ill patients are over-anxious to try new treatments, this is always difficult.

Eye Operations

The contact lens bandage in the form of the softer materials can be used to cover the eye at the end of the operation. This is particularly helpful after graft operations and may eventually be used in others too.

The complications following cataract surgery are rare but can lead to painful eyes. The use of soft and very large hard lenses can alleviate pain and in some instances give good vision.

Even these few examples are sufficient to give the reader some ideas of how plastics are used on and around the eye to help the surgeon in the treatment of disease.

Diagnostic Lenses

The ophthalmologist often wishes to know how well a diseased eye will see with contact lenses. For this purpose large optical lenses of several powers are kept. The tests are done with the comfort of local anaesthetic drops. The binocular vision can also be measured under these conditions.

The inside of the eye can be better examined by the use of special contact lenses. A special lens with a mirror included will allow the angle between the coloured portion and cornea to be minutely examined. The parts between the edge of the lens of the eye and the inner parts can also be seen. The retina of the eye can also be examined by such lenses.

The hard scleral lens can also be attached to electrodes and the type of electrical discharges from the eye accurately measured. Such information can be of great importance to assess the function of an eye and even the brain. It is not always necessary to take the electrical leads from the eye itself. The skull will often suffice. From such information even the type of sight a patient has can be measured.

Special lenses with metal inserts can be used to locate foreign bodies within the eye and orbit. The X-ray will not only show up the foreign body but its relationship to the marker contact lens.

Special Lenses and Uses

Swimmers often ask whether they can wear lenses under water. Certainly wearers of large hard lenses can. But all soft lenses may change their form and comfort if exposed to swimming pool water or very salty sea water. In general, small hard or soft lenses should be worn with under-water goggles and larger lenses only when the sea water has a low salt content.

To obtain magnification when the sight is poor a combination of contact lens and spectacles can be used. If the contact lens makes the eye a very weak power then the high power plus lens required in the spectacle correction will result in magnification. It is rarely a successful method of obtaining better sight. But the principle can be used to make two eyes even. This problem occurs after cataract operation on one eye when the contact lens correction results in abnormal image size.

The lids following severe burns caused by chemicals or heat may become adherent to the eye. In severe cases this can lead to blindness. The lids can be separated and kept separate for several weeks by the use of rings or contact lenses. This form of treatment can be very effective, but if there are insufficient tears, all will fail. In an effort to give the eyes a constant flow of tears, contact lenses and rings can be attached to capillary tubes feeding artificial tears fluid to the eye surface.

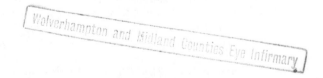

Chapter IX

MANUFACTURE OF CONTACT LENSES

Today we are accustomed to a very high expertise in technology. We also understand that production is concerned with manufacturing components to specifications. Such components will, when assembled, form complex pieces of machinery, the moon rocket being a supreme example. It must be realised that if even one vital component was not made to specification and not completely tested then the whole complex machine may fail. The contact lens is a one component article. Irrespective of how it is made and the material used, the end result must be according to specification. The testing of both the lens, basic material and solutions should conform to standards. Those standards are concerned with purity of materials, non-toxicity of the finished lens, both in materials and biological non-reaction, when on the eye. The optical finish must be such that good vision is possible. The tolerances allowed in manufacture must be very small, so that all lenses are reproduceable. The methods of measurement must be as accurate as the tolerances allowed in manufacture. Therefore methods of measuring the used lens must match those used by the manufacturer. Unless such a system exists, then the product becomes suspect and it is impossible for anyone to guarantee its properties within the tolerances acceptable for a good lens.

The layman may say what are those specifications? Can we know in what way they are critical and how do they affect the patient? To what degree of minuteness are the tolerances with which the manufacturer and practitioner have to work? Furthermore, solutions and drops used in contact lens wear must be considered in the same context because they can affect the lens and the eye.

The early contact lens of the 19th century described in the first chapter was large and made of glass. Its shape was measured by natural sight, and it was matched with a plaster model of an eye. Several lenses were made to form a set, and fitting was there-fore by trial and error. There were so many variables in eye curvature and size that good fitting by this method was more by luck than design. The power was ground on by equipment used to make large lenses (such as spectacles) and the results consider-ed crude when applied to small surfaces. Such contact lenses were the scleral (haptic) lenses, which fitted by touching the white of

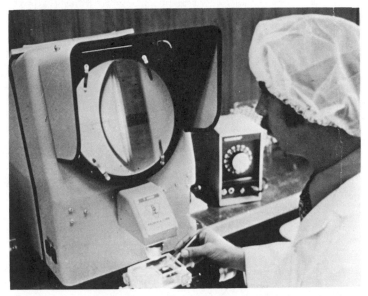

Fig. 34 Checking Quality (Photo Bausch & Lomb).

the eye but invariably formed a space between the cornea and front of the lens. Incidentally, such big lenses could be described in two parts, a central lens or optic portion, and an outer fitting or scleral portion. The scleral portion was eventually fitted by a moulding of the eye technique. Therefore the early contact lens was analogous to the spectacle lens. Whereas the spectacle lens was supported in front of the eye by the bridge of the nose and the ear, the contact lens was supported by the eye itself. In some instances by the white of the eye and in others by the cornea (the front window of the eye). The space between the back of the lens and the eye became filled with tear fluid and therefore the lens functioned optically slightly differently to the spectacle lens, which has air both in front and behind the lens. Furthermore, the optic of the lens moves with the eye.

The manufacturer can make such large lenses of many plastic or glass materials, but even if he produces a final result that is a good and accurate lens, there are several factors that are not under control and impossible to mention in the specification. Thus the lens has to be altered by a fitter to make it function. It is as if the components to a car were made so crudely that the assembler had to alter the parts to make them fit together. It is worthwhile mentioning these failings for a scleral lens because they are still used and the modern contact lenses applicable.

The model of the eye made of plaster from which the scleral lens is made may look like the eye in every detail, but is it the same size to a hundredth of a millimetre? One would discover that this may not be so. The plastic moulding material is porous, the surface soft and crumbly, and the wrinkles in the skin of the eye flattened out and the curvature of the cornea distorted by the technique. In other words, the technique of copying the eye is not exact enough to give us the accuracy we require in our specification. When we mould or inject contact lens plastic onto the plaster model, then more inaccuracies occur. Does the thin layer of plastic apply itself exactly to the plaster? Will it, after trimming and polishing, lens fitting and polishing and finally heating to body temperature, keep the original form to an accuracy of 1/100th. mm.? The answer is no. But is an accuracy required of 1/100th. mm.? The answer is yes. Because if the size of the lens varies, then the fit over the cornea will be fundamentally altered. Thus a large hat will, if it comes over the ears, come in contact with the top of the head, a small hat will touch the sides of the head and the top of the hat will stand clear of the head above. This analogy can be used for the eye. But whereas for the head the size tolerance may be $1''$ (2.5 cms.), for the eye it is measured in 1/100th mm. Therefore, if the manufacturer, is asked to prepare a scleral lens 1 mm. thick from a given model of the eye and told it must exactly fit the eye, he knows that it is impossible to copy the model and exactly fit the eye using present techniques. In the fitting of scleral lenses, the techniques used to overcome this failing were (see page 55) briefly mentioned.

Over ninety-nine per cent of the world's contact lens wearers use corneal lenses or hydrophilic scleral lenses. By definition, a corneal lens is one that essentially fits the cornea, and anything larger than the cornea having some fitting in the scleral portion is called a scleral lens. The sizes can vary within each definition. Thus the corneal lens can be as small as 7.00 and the smaller scleral 13 mm. in diameter, whereas the largest scleral can be 26 mm. in diameter depending upon the size of the eye. (See Chapter V.)

The materials are also interchangeable with the sizes. Thus a hydrophilic soft lens can be of corneal or scleral type, even though the majority of lenses commercially available are large lenses. The choice of fittings and materials will be described in the chapter upon fitting. In this chapter the technique used to manufacture preformed lenses will be described since it is this type that is used by the vast majority of patients. Preformed means that the shape is determined by geometrical specification and not individual shape of the eye. Given sufficient range of specifications and accuracy in manufacture, most lenses can be made to fit the eye without modification, the proviso being accurate measurements or use of materials or shapes that will conform or mould to a shape.

We remember that silk stockings were made in several sizes so that stress from a bad fit would not tear the fibres. Today the fibres used in stocking manufacture are stretchable and more elastic than silk for the same gauge. Therefore only two or three sizes to fit all shapes are necessary. The same process can be seen in contact lens practice. The harder materials are made to exact specifications of the eye shape and size, but soft elastic materials can be made to much wider tolerances and still give a satisfactory fitting.

The physical and chemical properties of the material will determine to a large extent the method of manufacture. For example, if a material can be heated and will at a certain temperature become fluid and, upon cooling, return to its former state without change, then such a material can be poured when hot into a mould and, when cool, become a contact lens or any other shape. To form the exact shape of the mould may require the help of pressure, either by air pressure spinning or casting. Some materials will not melt upon raising the temperature and this technique is not applicable. But many polymer plastics are formed by the interaction of monomers in a fluid state. Therefore it is possible to add a mixture of monomers in a fluid state to the mould and allow polymerization to take place. The set polymer will be a solid in the shape of the contact lens. Obviously I have over-simplified the process. There are many secrets in the process. It is exceedingly difficult to obtain a contact lens no thicker than 0.10 mm. in parts with regular optical geometrical surfaces, and high degree of homogenous (even) transparency. Such techniques, when perfected, are automatic and can result in many thousands of lenses being produced from the same moulds.

But the majority of lenses are produced by the use of a lathe. A lathe holds the raw material, in this case a button of plastic, at one end and holds a metal or diamond tool at the other. The button rotates at a high speed which must be consistent in speed and no jolting or irregularity in rotation is permissible. The chuck holding the button must grip firmly, so that at the beginning and at the end of the process no side movement whatsoever occurs of the button. It must be possible to control the setting of the button as to planes and position relative to the rotating spindle and therefore axis of the lathe. The best lathes have a very heavy base and fixed heavy tables or benches, so that no vibration will affect the setting of the button or diamond tool. The diamond must be cut in such a way that the point's angle is controllable and thé method of moving across the surface of the button related to this setting. The diamond must move evenly across the rotating button and describe a curvature measurable with accuracy. The accuracy we are speaking about is of the order of 2/100th. of a millimetre. By the use of a lathe, one or more spherical or toroidal surfaces can be cut on the back and front surfaces of the button, so making the basic contact lens. It is usual to cut the back surfaces first and then polish to produce an optical result. The button is then turned around and the front surfaces cut and polished, the thickness of the lens being controlled by the lathe settings.

Expertise in lathe work has enabled the manufacturer to form many alternative curvatures. The practitioner both at academic and practising levels is able to experiment to his heart's content. Using the eye shape as a model, fitting curvatures have been designed by many people from the simplest spherical forms to the most complex paraboloidal.

Irrespective of the way a lens is made, the perfection of finish and reproduceability of finish remain of paramount importance. The eye and lid surfaces recognise with painful results the sensation of rough or jagged surfaces. A comfortable lens must be examined every day before insertion just in case the material is wearing away or becoming damaged. A new lens may not feel the same as the old, even though all the measurements are accurate to 1/100th. mm. This proves, without doubt, that the parts of a lens not measurable, such as peripheral widths of curvature after the polishing process and quality of surface are very important to the wearer and practitioner.

Most of the materials used absorb water but some absorb almost 85% water and others as little as 1.4%. The absorption of water when over 2% results in a change in bulk. Thus a contact lens made of a dry plastic which absorbs 50% water will swell 20% in size. The manufacture of soft wet lenses is often by the technique of making a perfect small dry lens and then soaking it in saline or other physiological solution for several hours or even days. The lens will then have absorbed all the water it can. It should then be the correct power, curves and thickness required by the practitioner. Unfortunately, there are so many factors not completely under the control of the chemist and manufacturer that the final wet lens is seldom within the accuracy required. This has led to great problems in the development of soft lens practice. At present the methods of checking a soft wet lens are difficult. When better methods become available, more progress will be possible. Other workers say that since the water part of the lens is so variable and affected by temperature and salty content of tears and other chemical factors of the eye's function, it is impossible to set standards for measurement. To some extent this is true. The patient and practitioner must make some allowances for the manufacturer. He is often trying his best but the present plastics and methods of manufacture will not permit better reproduceability of the final lens.

To overcome these problems some manufacturers have made

their lathes automatic. The lathe is preset with all the required measurements and the entire process is then automatic. Unfortunately the polishing process which follows may not be so perfect and the gain in cutting accuracy may be lost.

There are several newer techniques used for special purposes. For example, lenses can be coloured by surface tinting, by inclusion (like a sandwich) of colour pigment, by inclusion of pigment or colour dyes uniformly in the material or in certain areas like a seaside rock. Such techniques also are applied to big scleral lenses.

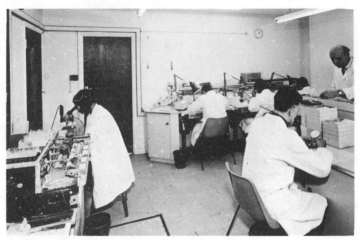

Fig. 35 Part of a laboratory making contact lenses (Photo/Hydron Ltd.).

Thus it is possible to make big scleral lenses look like an eye, the outer part being white with blood vessels and the inside coloured like the iris and pupil. Such appliances are used to make actor's eyes look abnormal or a different colour. The art of subterfuge is extensive and many bizarre appearances result. A fitter was once asked to make a pair of lenses for an actor to simulate severe damage done to the eyes. The result was so realistic that the close-up shots were not used.

The final lens is checked and labelled. All wet lenses should be made aseptic by either a chemical or heat method. They should then be packaged in a sterile container. Very often the lens and container are sterilised together. They will remain so until opened by the practitioner or patient.

Contact lens practice is now an industry but there still remain several patients seen each year that must be hand fitted. It is here that the manufacturer who works in mass production techniques becomes less useful.

The future may see the measurement of the vision and eye by photographic automated techniques. The results would then be computed and the lens manufacture determined by such results. Indeed such equipment is available although not applicable to all patients or eye conditions. It is indeed a pointer to the future unless knowledge advances and makes the need for appliances to correct vision just another stage in history.

Chapter X

QUESTIONS AND ANSWERS

Is there more than one type of lens?

There are three types of lens according to size. The large lens that covers the white is the scleral*; the one that completely covers the cornea the corneo-scleral, and the smallest is the corneal. *Sometimes called 'haptic'.

Are there variations for each type?

Yes, depending upon the principles applied for fitting or the standards adopted by the manufacturer.

Which is the correct type for my eye?

This decision rests with the practitioner.

Does the fitter have a philosophy that determines the best lens?

Yes, in brief the best lens is one that uses the minimal material but covers the maximal optical area; that can be worn for the longest time with the least damage to the eye tissues.

How many visits are necessary?

With the simplest lens a fitting, instruction and issue of lens could be done in one day, but it is often better to spread the visits so that 3 to 4 will end with the issue of lenses.

If I can wear my lenses comfortably, should I see my practitioner again?

It is unwise to wait until trouble arises before seeking advice. The practitioner should be consulted at regular intervals, either 6-monthly, yearly or two-yearly, according to their recommendation.

What will the practitioner determine at a routine visit?

If an ophthalmologist is seen, then any eye disease treatable will be assessed and diagnosed. All practitioners will evaluate the vision and the state of the contact lenses and eye. Optometrists will evaluate the normality of the eye and vision.

How can the patient know the status of the practitioner?
By the qualification:

Ophthalmologist —	M.B., B.S., M.R.C.S., L.R.C.P., L.S.A. Basic British Medical Qualifications.
	M.D. American Basic Medical Degree and British Higher Medical Degree.
	M.S. British Higher Degree in Surgery.
	D.O.M.S. Special Diploma in Ophthalmology.
	D.O. Special Diploma in Ophthalmology.
	F.R.C.S. (Oph.) Surgical Special. in Ophthalmology.
	M.D. Med. Specialist Oph. Continental Oph. Specialist.
Optometrist (or Ophthalmic Optician)	— D.O. American Degree in Optometry. B.Sc. (Oph. Optics). British Degree in Ophthalmic Optics.
	F.B.O.A. } British Professional Qualification for Ophthalmic F.S.M.C. } Opticians.
	D.C.L.P. Diploma in Contact Lens Practice.
Dispensing Optician	— Dispensing qualification of S.M.C. and B.O.A.
	F.A.D.O. — Fellow of Dispensing Opticians' Assn.
	Various Contact Lens Diplomas.

Are contact lens practitioners registrable?
Yes, a contact lens may only be supplied against a prescription given by a Medical Practitioner (Ophthalmologist) or an Optometrist. A Dispensing Optician may only fit and supply a contact lens under the supervision of an ophthalmologist or optometrist.

What is the difference between a Dispensing Optician and Ophthalmic Optician (optometrist)?
The Ophthalmic Optician is qualified to examine the eye. The Dispensing Optician is not. The Dispensing Optician may only fit

and supply appliances and cannot prescribe or give an opinion in any way to be interpreted as a diagnosis.

What is the difference between an Ophthalmologist and an Optometrist?

The Ophthalmologist is a medical specialist and can treat the patient by medical or surgical procedures. If they undertake to prescribe and fit contact lenses, then they are practising the optometric part of ophthalmology. If the contact lens is fitted as treatment of eye disease then it becomes a medical or surgical procedure.

Can contact lens practitioners advertise?

The medical contact lens specialist (ophthalmologist) must not advertise for patients in any form. The optometrists and dispensing opticians are allowed to advertise. It must be in a form acceptable to the General Optical Council.

How can I find the best practitioner?

In the same way as one would find the best solicitor or any other professional person. By asking one's friends, relatives, other contact lens wearers. Then by asking one's usual optical practitioner. If there is any doubt as to the normality of the eye, an opinion must be sought of a medical practitioner and/or ophthalmologist.

Is the fee charged by practitioners for contact lenses variable?

Yes. Very variable.

Why is this so?

The chief reason is that part of the fee is determined by the cost of the professional services of the practitioner. This will vary according to professional status and overheads. The contact lenses have a standard cost and some practitioners who manufacture lenses may be able to charge a minimal or *no* charge for the lenses. Thus an expert of high professional status working in an expensive area with technicians and having to pay the full cost of manufactured lenses may be charging two or three times the amount asked by a manufacturer who has established fitting clinics as a sideline.

How successful are contact lenses?

It depends on the expertise of fitting, the quality of manufacture and the tolerance and environment of the wearer. Providing everything is normal, 70% should be able to wear conventional corneal small thin lenses within one month. 90% should be able to wear softer materials. But if there are abnormalities, then failure may result with several types of lenses and after great expense.

How long do contact lenses last?

Hard low water content lenses can last indefinitely, but soft lenses wear out with constant and continued use. For some individuals they can wear out even after 3 months. The average time is $1\frac{1}{2}$ years. This will improve.

What care do lenses require over the years?

It is best to have new lenses as often as possible. About once every 3 years for hard lenses and every $1\frac{1}{2}$ for soft. Hard lenses can be repolished by special tools and re-edged. If done carefully and expertly, this will increase their comfort and life. But even so, once in a while the lens will warp with the treatment and become unwearable. The patient must take this risk if advised to have an old lens repolished.

Are there any laws or standards protecting the public against bad fitting or poor lenses?

There are laws which state indirectly the professional requirements of each body of practitioners. They do not specifically state contact lens practice. The medical specialists adhere to those standards advised by the General Medical Council and the optical practitioners by the General Optical Council. The standards of teaching are controlled by many departments, both government professional bodies and university. The optical bodies award diplomas in expertise for contact lens fitting practice. There are no standards in the U.K. for quality of materials, solutions or manufacture, but the Medicine Acts will soon formulate regulations. In the U.S.A. the F.D.A. has formulated a series of phases for the examination of materials and lenses to be worn by the public. It is a lengthy and very expensive process but protects the public.

Should I experience pain when wearing contact lenses?

No, only if dust or foreign bodies become lodged behind the lens or if you inadvertently damage the eye, or if the lens is worn too long or under bad conditions against the practitioner's advice.

What are the do's and don'ts for the hard lens wearer beginning to adapt?

(1) Make sure hands are clean and no make-up on eyes.
(2) The lenses are prepared as recommended or washed and wetted.
(3) Give as much time as necessary for learning insertion and removal *before* commencing wear.
(4) Commence to wear when fresh and not fatigued.
(5) Commence wear with increased blinking rate.
(6) Have good ventilation present. Avoid smoky, dusty and windy atmospheres in the early stages.
(7) Commence with 2 to 4 hours and add 1 hour daily until up to 10 hours, then seek advice about wearing time.
(8) Observe practitioner's advice regarding alternative build-up times, since lenses have individual properties.
(9) Clean lenses after removal and store as recommended.

Is it best to keep hard lenses in solution or dry?

If lenses are being kept for long periods without being worn, such as spare lenses, then dry storage is least problematic.

Most lenses to be worn daily should be stored in the *correct* solution.

N.B. Some solutions are only to be used for *hard* lenses and must not be used for *soft*.

What is the best way to clean and disinfect soft wet lenses?

Each manufacturer suggests their own best method. Most recommend heating in normal salt solution (or a special 'buffered' salt solution). There are solutions for storage but the practitioner must advise. There are enzyme and other cleaning agents for soft lenses to remove sticky materials from the surfaces. They should be used as often as necessary. For the average person once a week is sufficient, but for others with good tear function once a month may be advised.

Can I sleep with my lenses on?

Some types of lenses can be slept with but most hard types *must* be removed.

What are the consequences of sleeping with lenses?

For some patients, especially if deficient of tears and if hard lenses are worn, the reaction can be severe with pain and blurred sight, even requiring hospital treatment.

Should I have red eyes even after wearing contact lenses for 5 years?

Most contact lenses cause a reaction. This results in increased size and number of blood vessels in the lids and white of the eye. Stopping contact lens wear may not reverse the redness to complete normality.

What is the treatment for redness of eyes with good contact lens tolerance?

A smaller thinner lens, or softer material, may be advised.

What forms of insurance are available?

Normal all-risks insurance can be obtained to cover loss and breakage of contact lenses. The sum to insure for is the replacement cost. This is much less than the initial cost of lenses.

e.g. Consultations
Fitting and Supply of Lenses	= £85.00 (170 $)
Replacement cost	= £20.00 (40 $) per lens

There are other forms of insurance which are only available from specialist firms or the manufacturer. Read the clauses carefully. They vary considerably. Insurance does not usually cover spoilage or wear and tear of lenses and it does not cover new lenses required if the power changes.

Are drops useful when wearing contact lenses?

Yes, several types of drops can be used as lubricants. Many contain no drugs and can be used as often as necessary. Drug-containing drops can only be prescribed by a medical practitioner (or ophthalmologist). They may be prescribed to treat infection or reduce inflammation. Special advice is necessary if using drops with wet soft lenses.

Do contact lenses improve the sight?

In the early stages slight swelling of the corneal surface will result in blurred vision, especially at night or if spectacles are worn. Some patients after several years' wear develop slight curvature changes of the eye with improvement of sight. The incidence of severe scarring or infection is less than normal eye disease and will not occur for the normal eye. It will occur if the eyes are diseased before contact lens wear begins.

Are there any ethical agreements between practitioners?

No, but many practitioners belong to the same societies and will conform to basic ethics.

> e.g. They will not treat another practitioner's patient without consent.
> They will send a report of their findings.
> They will attempt to reconcile aggrieved or intolerant patients to their original practitioner.
> They will refer patients for specialist opinions whenever necessary.

For intolerance cases that occur within 6 months of commencing wear the lenses will be taken back if in good condition and a proportion of the cost returned to the patient. If a patient has not expended all the professional services portion of the fee, then a proportion also will be returned.

If I go to a contact lens practitioner for advice but do not go ahead with a fitting or am not advised to have contact lenses, do I have to pay a fee?

Yes, for professional advice.

Will contact lenses be fitted by the present technique in the foreseeable future?

The fitting and prescribing may become separate to the dispensing. The latter may eventually become an over-the-counter transaction of a sealed guaranteed package obtainable only on prescription. In some countries this is enforced for ethical reasons.

Can I obtain contact lenses from the N.H.S.*?

Only if advised by a hospital ophthalmologist. In most instances the need for contact lenses will only be considered on clinical grounds and not upon aesthetic, cosmetic or occupational factors.

Do contact lenses correct squints?

If the squint is associated with long-sight and abnormality of using close vision, then contact lenses will correct the squint just the same as spectacles. If the squint is of a different type, they will not correct the squint. In such cases spectacles have a better cosmetic masking effect.

Can I swim and sunbathe with contact lenses?

In general, the eyes that wear contact lenses are more sensitive to glare and sunlight, therefore dark glasses are advised as a protective. For swimming underwater or in rough sea only large well-fitted scleral can be worn with safety. Corneal hard and soft lenses can be used in combination with a pair of goggles (snorkel type). Soft lenses may absorb the swimming pool water and alter their fitting and result in irritation and loss.

Do contact lenses protect the eyes against injury?

Yes, they act as a protective layer against foreign bodies or chemicals. But if the remainder of the eye is injured, the presence of the contact lens can cause further irritation. In the presence of flash (arc) or flying metal foreign bodies, protective goggles or spectacles must be worn.

Are contact lenses experimental?

Yes, they are continuing to change in material and design. All commercially available lenses are of proven design and, if tolerance is good, need not be changed until advised. As with most manu-factured articles, depending upon advanced technology, improvements are introduced yearly.

*National Health Service.

Chapter XI

CORRECTION OF SIGHT BY OTHER METHODS

In order that the reader should obtain the correct perspective this chapter will outline the conventional, non-conventional and experimental methods of correcting defective eyesight. It has already been indicated that good vision develops very soon after birth and if insufficient stimulus for sight is present within even the first few months of life, then defective sight may result. The analysis of the type of defect using normal examination methods and then, where necessary, more elaborate techniques is important before commencing treatment.

Spectacles are an inexpensive and accurate way of correcting most power defects of the eye. If worn from an early age they will help develop good vision. If the power defect is large and present at birth, then other methods besides spectacles have to be tried. Contact lenses as an alternative have been described. Irrespective of the external optical methods used, if the nervous system serving the eyesight is also defective, then good vision will not be possible. Future research and clinical assessment will be directed towards techniques that can establish the expectations of vision for patients with eye and brain abnormalities as early as possible in life. Treatment will then be directed towards giving the best optical correction as soon as possible. Whilst a baby may have some difficulty in wearing spectacles and, surprisingly enough, less with contact lenses, the future may see the use of other methods.

There are many treatments for correcting vision where spectacles or contact lenses are not used. Some methods are exercises, others drugs. Some treatments are really experimental and involve the use of appliances and surgery not generally known to the public. They are not without risk and therefore the public must still consider them to a degree experimental.

Diet has been thought to be a cause of short-sightedness. Some races are essentially vegetarian, others carnivorous. There are races where famine and taboos exclude the use of specific dietary essentials. The summation of this knowledge has led investigators to suggest that low protein diet in early infancy and even puberty may result in an eye that is short-sighted. The exact mechanism is not known and the results not fully collaborated by other research workers. Irrespective of its value, if protein deficiency is diagnosed or incomplete diet, then supplementary foods or a new diet is given. It must be realised that in most instances a measurable degree of short-sight has occurred before treatment is even considered. Such a degree of short-sight may be non-progressive anyway. Whilst most medical treatments are instituted to delay or prevent further development, very few can correct the short-sight already established. There are exceptions to this. For example, sugar diabetes can, if not treated, result in defects of sight, the commonest being short-sightedness. Once treatment has established normal sugar metabolism then the eyesight returns to normal. One thinks that the change in sight was due to the lens of the eye swelling with increased water. However, changes in the eye tissue due to diabetes but unrelated to water cannot be corrected by treatment and return to normality. Even with modern laser techniques where leaking blood vessels at the back of the eye are sealed, the aim of treatment is always to prevent further complications from occurring not unfortunately to restore normality.

The Eskimos knew that if the eye lids could be closed to a slit better vision resulted and glare from the snow decreased. They even invented some thousand years ago wooden bars with slits to produce the same effect. These spectacles are still available in modern form. They look like spectacles but have horizontal slits. Another type is multiple holes. Each hole will allow light to reach the eye and form an image at the back of the eye which is narrow enough not to require power modifications and still permit good vision. Such methods reduce the brilliance of the image and also drastically reduce the field, but where all optical appliances fail, they provide an inexpensive last resort that will give some comfort.

We are advised by some authorities, mostly non-medical, to

exercise our eye muscles, so that the shape can be naturally modified and so correct vision. Such techniques may also involve control of accommodation and use the narrowed palpebral fissure. It is unusual for such methods to correct sight more than 1 to 2 units. Since they are advised and practised by non-registered practitioners, their value is suspect. They have been in use for more than a century but no scientific appraisal of the methods has been made. Their true value is doubtful.

Certainly excessive reading can cause a spasm of accommodation, so that the focus stops for near sight. The eyesight cannot relax for distance. Thus students and young persons who are always at close quarters with their work can suffer from this form of induced myopia. Stopping their studies and introducing outdoor activities daily can make the eyesight return to normal. It is possibly a good idea to make all persons, young and old, mix their activities and work so that constant close focus is avoided. With this in mind and for other good philosophical reasons, we should all be able to escape from our tasks to use the body and mind in a different way as often as possible. The western civilisation has much to learn from the east in this respect.

In a more positive way drugs, such as atropine, are used in the eye to paralyse the muscle that makes the lens change its power. By this technique short-sight of up to -1.50 units can be neutralized. Whilst some authorities claim that this method used in children will cure small degrees of short-sight, it is by no means proven. The child, furthermore, has the inconvenience of wearing spectacles for reading and suffering light sensitivity problems throughout the period of treatment. It is in this group of patients that further research may clarify how short-sight develops and to what degree each child may be affected.

It may be relevant here to discuss briefly the use of optical corrections for children with squint since it is intimately connected with the development of vision. The human being can use both eyes together almost from birth. Certainly in a more primitive way for the whole field of vision and with focusing for the critical and acute vision. Unfortunately some babies are born with visual obstacles which prevent the two eyes working together. For example, the brain may be deficient in the mechanism for making the two eyes work together, or the nerves and muscles which manipulate the two eyes may be damaged or deficient. The eyes, themselves, may be abnormal and therefore unable to receive the high quality pictures that the brain requires to superimpose and fuse into one stereoscopic picture. One of the commonest causes is the presence of power abnormalities. It has been said that if the eyes could be corrected early enough, then they would function and good vision would develop. Furthermore, if one eye is not being used, it can be encouraged by covering the good eye. In very young people such treatment must be very carefully supervised, otherwise the normal eye itself can become weak if covered too long. Without suitable tests for babies and children much depends on what the parents have to report about eye function. The ability of the child to find and play with very small coloured objects can be used as a method of testing sight. Such methods take a long time to evaluate, but the truth is that without good optical correction the other treatments are limited. Even the operations to straighten eyes may have limited results if the eyes cannot function normally as far as the sight is concerned.

The development of abnormal sight in infancy, puberty or young adult is usually due to myopia. Whilst the smaller degrees can be blamed upon either heredity or to excessive reading, the more progressive types resulting in high degrees and changes at the back of the eye must be considered an inborn error and so far not treatable. Experimental work tends to show that high temperature with fever may cause myopia to develop or that increased pressure in the eye due to anatomical or physiological inborn abnormalities may also be a cause, but there is no proof. One cannot prevent or treat conditions that are still of hypothetical origin.

In an effort to strengthen the eye muscles, especially the outside ones controlling the lids, some practitioners have used galvanic current stimulation. Others have tried stimulating the neck where nerves are known to emerge. Yet others believe in acupuncture, psychoanalysis or even hypnosis. It is obvious that where the cause of defective sight is not known a host of treatments is available. They are often suggested by sincere practitioners and accepted by over-anxious patients or parents. The results based upon scientific principles remain problematical.

Surgical Procedures

Man has designed many operations based upon mechanical principles to correct power problems. They must all be considered experimental. No patient would be submitted to such methods of treatments unless their condition could not be treated by other methods. The ethics controlling these procedures vary according to the professional attitudes and regulations of each country. Most communities require the patient to volunteer for such operations and waive any responsibility of outcome so as to clear the practitioner.

Short-sight of high degree can be corrected by shortening the eye. This is done by removing a strip of eye tissue at the equator and then sewing the eye up. The cornea can be made a flatter curve. This can be done be incisions. It can also be done by taking the front of the cornea off the eye, freezing it to make it hard, cutting a different curve on a lathe and then sewing it back to the eye. The cornea thus has a loss of power and is thinner. This can accurately correct high degrees of short-sight but is not without dangers.

The curvature of the cornea can be permanently flattened by surgical techniques but they all involve injury to the cornea and therefore the possibility of infection or even distorted vision from abnormal scar reaction. Operations to increase the curvature of the cornea and so add power to the eye are more limited. One operation inserts a small lens made of human cadaver cornea. The small lens increases the thickness of the cornea at the centre and steepens the curvature. This operation is sometimes done to correct high degrees of long-sight after cataract extraction, but because of its complexity and unknown results, it would not be recommended as routine procedure.

The contact lens, itself, can be fitted in such a way as to mould the cornea to a new shape. Not sufficient work has been done on infants' cornea to establish whether this can occur permanently. Very often changes in curvature, if permanent, are associated with scar tissue forming in the cornea and distortion of vision.

There are several bizarre operations concerned with placing plastic lenses on the cornea, in the cornea, in the eye itself, some of which have become routine procedures.

Several years ago it was found that the surface skin of the cornea, if removed, provided a base to which a contact lens could be adhered thus giving a permanent contact lens. The results proved such lenses to be wearable for 2 years or more and are still used in the treatment of gross water logging of the cornea. This is a serious disease and no other simple procedures can correct the sight so well, but for the correction of normal sight the adhesive is too toxic and results in complications.

A nut and bolt made of plastic with the bolt part performing an optical function and the nut a fixing device was designed. It required the cornea to be cut into and the lens removed. In some eyes such appliances had a limited life and the complications could be severe. Other similar operations can be done but the consensus of opinion is to leave them for very rare cases. They are not used routinely.

After the cataract is removed, some surgeons insert a small plastic lens which remains in the eye permanently. There can, of course, be complications and if the patient elects to have this operation, the risk factor must be understood. The results have proven to be very good and are especially valuable in elderly persons who would find spectacles or contact lenses difficult to manage.

One hopes that future methods of correcting vision will have no complications; that if possible with increased knowledge the causes of defective vision will be better understood and their control and treatment possible by medical techniques rather than by optical or surgical procedures. That time will be in the far distance. Until then for the average person spectacles and contact lenses must suffice.

INDEX

Albinos, contact lenses for, 68
Allergy to eye drops, 58
Aphakia, correction with contact
     lenses, 38, 68
Astigmatism, 15
Atmosphere for contact lens wear,
     58

Bending light power (B.L.P.), 25
Bifocal lenses, 65
Brain, visual centre, 16, 17
Burns, corneal, 58

Children, optical corrections for
     squint, 90
Cleaning agents, 53
Complications, 56–65
     optical, 63
Conoid lenses, 40
Contact lenses, bifocal, 65
     cost, 33
     curve, checking, 47
     durability, 83
     fitting, 41–55
     hypermobility, 64
     invention, 1–5
     manufacture, 28–29, 72–79
     removal, 54
     sight correction by, 21–26
     types, 80
     water absorption, 77
     weight, 21
Contraceptives, oral, effect on
     contact lens wear, 59
Cornea, action on light rays, 23

cells, 11
curvature, 12
distortion, 64
function, 10
oedema, 64
scarring, effects, 15
ulcers, 59
water logging, 93
Corneal lenses, materials for, 39
     sizes, 38, 39
Corneo-scleral lenses, 37
     materials for, 39
Cost of contact lenses, 33

Diagnostic lenses, 44, 45, 70
Diagnostic unit, 45
Diet, effect on vision, 89
Discomfort, 57
Drug dispensation by contact
     lenses, 66
Dust, 57

Eye, abnormal, contact lenses for,
     68
     diseases, treatment with contact
          lenses, 66–71
     disfigured, contact lenses for, 68
     drops, 85
     dry, treatment with contact
          lenses, 69
     focusing, 15
     function, 6–20
     implants, 69
     internal, examination with
          contact lens, 70

lens, 15
muscles, strengthening methods, 91
plaster model, 74
plastic implants, 92
powers, abnormal, correction with contact lenses, 66
errors, 14
variation, types, 13
structure, 7
surgical procedures, 92
contact lens bandage, 70
Eyelids, burns, treatment with contact lens support, 71
discomfort, 63

Fees, 33, 82
Fit assessment, 45
Fitting of contact lenses, 41–55
Fluorescent dye test of fit, 45
Focimeter, 48
Focusing, 15

Gels, hydrophilic, soft, 24
Glare, 64

Haptic contact lenses, 35
Hard contact lenses, 35, 84
History of contact lenses, 1–5
Holes in lenses, 40
Hypermetropia, 15

Infection, 62
Insertion of lens, 51–53
Insurance, 85
Intermediate lenses, 37

Keratoconus, correction with contact lenses, 67
treatment, surgical, 92

Legislation, protective, 83
Lens, artificial, 93
crystalline, 15
curve, checking, 47
Lubricants, 49, 55, 89

Magnification with contact lenses and spectacles, 71
Manufacture of lenses, 28–29, 72–79
Materials for contact lenses, 21
Menstruation and contact lens wear, 59
Multi-image formation, 64
Multispherical lenses, 40
Myopia, 15, 49, 91

National Health Service, lenses supplied under, 33, 87
Non-round lenses, 40

Ophthalmic and Dispensing optician role in lens fitting, 31
Ophthalmologist, role in lens fitting, 29
Optic nerves, 16
Oxygen lack, 59

Pain due to contact lenses, 84
Perspex, 4
physical properties, 21–23
Plastics, 4
implants, 92
water-adsorbing, 24
Polymethyl methacrylate, 21
Practitioner's role, 27–34
Practitioners, registration, 81
Pregnancy and contact lens wear, 59
Prism lenses, 40
Pseudo-conoidal lenses, 40

Radiuscope, 47
Red eyes, 62
Removal of lenses, 54
Retina, sensitivity, 6

Saline solution, 49
Scleral contact lenses, 3, 4, 35
advantages, 36
contraindications, 37
material for, 37

Sensitivity to lenses, 56
Silicon rubber, 24
Skin disorders affecting eye, 59
Sleep with contact lenses, 85
Soft lens, 37, 42, 43, 45, 84
Squint, correction with contact
    lenses, 87
    optical correction, 90
Sterilisation and Disinfection, 84
    kit, 54
Storage, 53
Sunlight and contact lenses, 87
Surgical procedures, 92
Swimming with contact lenses, 71,
    87

Tear fluid, 22, 42
Tears, abnormal, and contact lens
    wear, 59

Trial lenses, 44, 45
Tuohy, 5

Ulcers, corneal, 59

Vision, binocular, 19
    cerebral localisation, 16, 17
    clouding, due to contact lenses,
        63
    double, 65
    stereoscopic, 18
    variations, 13

Water adsorption by contact lens,
    77
Water-adsorbing plastics, 24
Watery haze due to tears, 64
Weight of contact lens, 21